REBUILD YOUR BRAIN:

Stop the Damage
Start the Repair

DR. BEN GALYARDT, D.C.

Dedication

This book is dedicated to my wife Michelle, whose every health challenge has propelled me into another phase of healing for others. To my parents Dennis and Amy and brother Wes who have been there for me throughout my life in any form that was needed. To all of my mentors and teachers that I've been blessed to learn from; Walter, Mark, Ian, Craig, Dietrich, Andy, Isaac, Frankie, Richard, and Datis. And most importantly my four boys; Dylan, Rohan, River, and Gavyn, who motivate me every day to keep my brain working optimally.

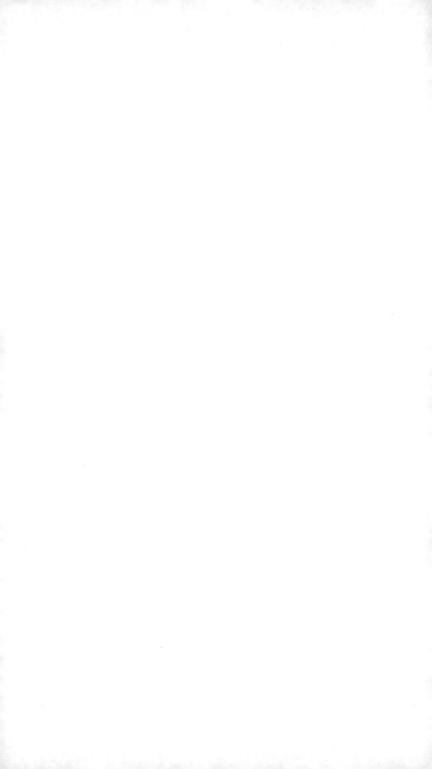

TABLE OF CONTENTS

ABOUT THE AUTHOR

"My purpose on this planet is to help empower others to optimize their bodies health, so they can contribute more to humanity and to live full, healthy lives."

-Dr. Ben Galyardt

Dr. Galyardt is a world recognized speaker in *Neurofeedback and Brain Regeneration*. He coaches doctors all over the country on how to help their patients find their highest potential and obtain optimal health.

Dr. Galyardt's Board Certifications, Degrees and Training include:

- *Board Certified in Integrative Medicine*
- *Certified Neurofeedback Practitioner*
- *International College Applied Kinesiology (AK)*
- *Neuro-Emotional Technique (NET) Certification*
- *Trigenics Practitioner*
- *Certified by the American Functional Neurology Institute*
- *Advanced Muscle Integration Technique (AMIT)*
- *Autonomic Response Testing (ART) by Dr. Dietrich Klinghardt*
- *Bachelors from Syracuse University in Health and Exercise Science*
- *Graduated from Parker College of Chiropractic in Dallas, Texas*

CHAPTER 1

Your Brain Can Heal

"There is no scientific study more vital to man than the study of his own brain. Our entire view of the universe depends on it."

~ FRANCIS H.C. CRICK (FROM SCIENTIFIC AMERICAN, SEPTEMBER 1979)

"You are constantly growing new brain cells into your 50s, 60s, 80s, and 90s – throughout your lifetime – through a process called neurogenesis."

~ DAVID PERLMUTTER

According to conventional medical wisdom, each person is born with a fixed number of brain cells. Until the last 15-20 years, neuroscientists believed that the brain did not have the ability to heal; it could not repair itself or grow new cells. So if any brain cells were damaged, they were permanently lost.

However, recent research has proved that the brain can create new cells (**neurogenesis**) as well as new pathways (**synaptogenesis**) throughout life. There is a continuous process of degeneration and regeneration of brain cells. When this process becomes imbalanced, we see more degeneration. Then we need to slow down the damage and speed up the regeneration to truly heal the brain.

This process is similar to that of degeneration and regeneration in bones. Bone cells are being continuously broken down and rebuilt. Osteoclasts break down old bone, while at the same time, osteoblasts are building up new bone. When this balance is altered, that is, either the breaking down is faster, or the building up is slower, it can lead to osteoporosis.

Researchers at Cornell University Medical College in New York City demonstrated that brain cells from a part of the brain called the hippocampus can continue to divide and grow in a laboratory dish. The hippocampus plays an important role in learning, memory, and quality of memories. These cells were taken from patients undergoing surgery to repair brain disorders.

This research proves that, given the right tools, the brain can regenerate around the damaged areas. Up to 700 neurons per day can be replaced in the hippocampus. That is like replacing the entire hippocampus by the time we turn 50.

This could lead to restoring diseased and damaged cells in the hippocampus and other regions of the brain. Ultimately, it raises the hope of treating degenerative brain diseases such as Parkinson's and Alzheimer's.[1]

The ability of the brain to create new neurons and new connections, and to reorganize neural pathways is called **neuroplasticity** or **brain plasticity**.

There are two types of neuroplasticity:

Functional Plasticity is the brain's ability to move functions from a damaged area of the brain to other undamaged areas. This movement of functions even comes from the opposite side of the brain.

Structural Plasticity is the brain's ability to change its physical structure as a result of learning. This can be strengthening the existing cells or generating new cells.

Both genetics and environment may have a role to play in neuroplasticity. For example, when you are learning a new skill, the more you practice it, the better you become. This is because your brain forms new neural pathways in response to your efforts. On the other hand, your brain eliminates the pathways that you no longer use.

Neuroplasticity applies to emotional states as well. For example, if you are anxious, your neural pathways become wired for anxiety. If you learn how to be calm, those anxiety pathways are progressively reduced. This is seen many times when a brain map (QEEG) is performed on someone who has learned to meditate and has practiced it for years. Their map shows a much slower electrical activity in the areas of the brain that are related to anxiety, rumination, and obsessive thoughts.

The U.S. government launched the BRAIN Initiative in 2013 to "revolutionize our understanding of the human mind."[2]

- The goals of this program are to understand:
- patterns of neural activity that produce cognition
- how brain activity leads to perception, decision-making and ultimately action
- how information is stored and processed in neural networks
- mysteries of normal and abnormal brain function
- mysteries of brain disorders such as Alzheimer's and Parkinson's diseases, depression, post-traumatic stress disorder (PTSD), and traumatic brain injury[3]

Five Science-Backed Ways to Strengthen Your Brain

Here are five simple daily habits to stimulate neuroplasticity and boost your brain power:

1. Eat Healthy Food

What you eat plays a crucial role in protecting and promoting the functioning of your brain. Avoid sugar and processed foods and eat more fresh vegetables. Also, there is a close connection between the microbes in your gut (microbiome) and your brain. Probiotic supplements or fermented vegetables that provide high levels of beneficial bacteria can help to improve brain function.

2. Exercise Regularly

During exercise, the brain releases neurotrophic factors such as BDNF (brain-derived neurotrophic factor), which improve brain functions, helps repair damaged neurons and encourages the growth of new neurons in the brain. The most effective exercise is high-intensity interval exercise (HIIT), even performed 1-2 times per week can increase BDNF significantly. Other recommended exercises include swimming, Pilates, yoga, strength training, and brisk walking. A sedentary lifestyle is an independent risk factor for cardiac disease, and premature death. So, you also need to be active throughout the day.

3. Get Proper Sleep

All of us have experienced the effects of lack of sleep on the brain. During the quality sleep state, referred to as the Delta state, the body will repair and rebuild many tissues in the body, especially brain tissue. Regular good-quality sleep is crucial for neural functions such as learning, memory, and neuroplasticity. Many people worry about the length that they are sleeping but the more important factor is the quality of that sleep. For even greater benefit, take a short mid-day nap. Even 20 minutes is sufficient to refresh the mind and improve productivity.

4. Stimulate Your Mind

Become a lifelong student and commit to learning something new repeatedly. As already explained, engaging in "cognitively demanding" activities helps to stretch and expand all function of the brain such as memory, focus, learning, and so on.

When someone asks about crossword puzzles or Sudoku or Luminosity, I tell them they are fine to keep their mind active but it won't have a significant amount of neural stimulation. Learning a new skill is much more demanding on the brain and it will respond with dramatic growth.

A 2015 study of people aged 85 and older published in Neurology showed that those who used a computer late in life and engaged in artistic and social activities had a lower risk of mild cognitive impairment.[4]

5. Develop a Positive Attitude

Your attitude about life is the most important factor in maintaining a strong brain. A positive attitude includes developing positive mental qualities such as cheerfulness, gratitude, compassion, empathy, forgiveness, and goodwill. It also includes practices such as mindfulness and generosity. An optimistic outlook also helps to improve your general health and quality of life.

References

1. WebMD. (2000, March 6). Get Smart: Brain Cells Do Regrow, Study Confirms. Retrieved from http://www.webmd.com/brain/news/20000306/get-smart-brain-cells-do-regrow-study-confirms#1

2. National Institute of Mental Health. (2013). Multimedia about BRAIN Initiative. Retrieved from https://www.nimh.nih.gov/news/media/index-brain-initiative.shtml

3. Dr. Mercola. (2015, June 11). Neurosurgeon Reflects on the Awe and Mystery of the Brain. Retrieved from http://articles.mercola.com/sites/articles/archive/2015/06/11/brain-mysteries.aspx

4. Roberts R.O. et al. (2015, May 5.) Risk and protective factors for cognitive impairment in persons aged 85 years and older. Neurology, 84, 18, 1854-61.

CHAPTER 2

Neurodegeneration

"True ignorance is not the absence of knowledge, but the refusal to acquire it."

~ KARL POPPER

*"Ashes to ashes
Dust to dust
Oil those brains
Before they rust."*

~ J. PRELUTSKY

Neurodegeneration is the gradual deterioration in a person's cognitive abilities, such as memory, perception, judgment, and learning. This loss is due to either death of neurons or structural changes that prevent their normal functioning.

Breakdown of nerve cells in the brain happens regularly and is part of the healthy functioning of the brain. To work optimally the brain needs to remove old cells that are no longer serving their purpose and build new cells to take their place. It is when this process gets out of balance with not enough building or too much breakdown that we see the decline in brain function.

Neurodegeneration is the main feature of neurodegenerative diseases such as Alzheimer's disease, vascular dementia, Parkinson's disease, amyotrophic lateral sclerosis (ALS), and Huntington's disease. There are many other reasons why a loss of brain cells occurs in the body and we will delve into many of these reasons throughout this book.

Causes of neurodegeneration

About five percent of neurodegenerative diseases are due to genetic mutations. The remaining cases may be caused by the accumulation of toxic proteins in the brain or defective functioning of brain mitochondria and creation of toxic molecules.[1]

NEURODEGENERATIVE DISEASES

1. Dementia

Dementia affects memory, thinking, behavior, and the ability to perform everyday activities. It is classified as a major neurocognitive disorder because it interferes with both cognitive function and performing everyday activities. Cognitive function includes memory, language, speech, reasoning, judgment, and other thinking abilities.

Different causes of dementia are associated with distinct symptoms and brain abnormalities. Many people, especially those in the older age groups, may have more than one cause of dementia, which is called mixed dementia.

Some conditions that mimic dementia are thyroid disorders, depression, delirium, vitamin deficiencies, chronic alcoholism, and side effects from medications. Unlike dementia, these conditions may be reversed by appropriate treatment.

2. Alzheimer's disease

About 5.4 million Americans have Alzheimer's disease, and it is the sixth leading cause of death in the United States.

Alzheimer's disease is a degenerative brain disease and the most common cause of dementia. In Alzheimer's disease, the damage and destruction of neurons eventually affect other parts of the brain. Alzheimer's disease is ultimately fatal. Early symptoms include difficulty recalling recent conversations, names or events as well as depression and apathy. Later symptoms include impaired communication, disorientation, confusion, poor judgment, behavior changes and, ultimately, difficulty speaking, swallowing and walking.[2]

The main features of Alzheimer's disease are the progressive accumulation of beta-amyloid plaques outside neurons in the brain and twisted tau strands (tangles) inside neurons. These changes lead to damage and death of the affected neurons. Research is showing that many cases of Alzheimer's are caused by elevated sugar in the body. This is the main reason that researchers are calling it Type 3 diabetes.

No single test can diagnose Alzheimer's disease. Instead, a variety of approaches and tools have to be used to make a diagnosis including medical and family history, cognitive tests, and physical and neurologic examinations.

No medication that slow or stops the progression of Alzheimer's disease. The FDA has approved six drugs to alleviate symptoms of Alzheimer's disease: galantamine, rivastigmine, donepezil, memantine, tacrine and a drug that combines memantine and donepezil. (Tacrine has been discontinued in the U.S. due to severe side effects.) However, none of these drugs slows or stops the progression of Alzheimer's disease.[2]

Other measures include exercise, memory training, neurofeedback, art therapy, activity-based therapy, and activities such as gardening, cooking, word games, and listening to music may be helpful. Neurofeedback may help to reduce mild cognitive impairment, which is usually the first stage of Alzheimer's disease.[2]

3. Vascular dementia

Vascular dementia is responsible for ten percent of dementia cases. Vascular dementia is caused by the blockage or damage of blood vessels leading to infarcts or bleeding in the brain. Their number, size, and location determine the extent and symptoms of dementia. Impaired ability to make decisions is the first symptom. Other symptoms include slow gait and poor balance.[2]

4. Parkinson's disease

Nearly one million people in the US are living with Parkinson's disease, a chronic and progressive movement disorder (including slowness, rigidity, tremor, and changes in gait). In Parkinson's disease, neurons in an area of the brain called the substantia nigra are damaged. This leads to decreased production of dopamine, which controls movement and coordination.

The hallmark sign of Parkinson's disease is the presence of clumps of a protein called alpha-synuclein. There is presently no cure for Parkinson's disease. However, its symptoms can be managed with the help of medications and other measures. Vast amounts of research have come out in the last couple of years showing the connection between imbalances in the microbiome and Parkinson's disease.

5. Amyotrophic lateral sclerosis (ALS, Lou Gehrig's disease)

ALS is a progressive neurodegenerative disease that affects nerve cells in the brain and the spinal cord. Amyotrophic means "no muscle nourishment." When a muscle doesn't get nourishment, it wastes away. «Lateral» identifies the location of the nerve cells that control the muscles in the spinal cord. When these cells degenerate, it causes hardening («sclerosis»). The nerves that are affected in ALS are the motor neurons that provide voluntary movements and muscle control. With voluntary muscle action progressively affected, patients in the later stages of the disease may become totally paralyzed.

There is one FDA approved drug, riluzole, which slows the progression of ALS in some people. According to the American Academy of Neurology's Practice Parameter Update, participation in a multidisciplinary ALS clinic may prolong life and improve its quality.[2]

6. Huntington's disease

Huntington's disease is an inherited disease that causes the progressive breakdown of neurons in the brain. This brain damage gets progressively worse and impairs thinking, movement, and behavior. There's no cure for Huntington's disease and its progress cannot be reversed or slowed down. Medication can help to reduce some of the symptoms.

Currently, there is no cure for neurodegeneration, though there are specific drugs that can be used to minimize their symptoms, such as L-dopa for Parkinson's, riluzole for ALS, and so on. A healthy diet, exercise and cognitive engagement, such as brain games and learning new skills, can help reduce the symptoms of neurodegeneration and delay its onset.

Early detection of these neurodegenerative disorders is crucial. Consult your doctor if you notice signs such as abnormal changes in your memory, slurred speech, muscle weakness, and tremors in the hands or feet and so on.

References

1. Ontario Brain Institute. (n.d.) Brainnovation Snapshot. Retrieved from http://www.braininstitute.ca/sites/default/files/neurodegeneration_brainnovation_final.pdf

2. Alzheimer's Association. (2016.) 2016 Alzheimer's Disease Facts and Figures. Retrieved from https://www.alz.org/documents_custom/2016-facts-and-figures.pdf

CHAPTER 3

Traumatic Brain Injury

"As the mother of a grown son with a traumatic brain injury, I couldn't be more excited about the prospect of finding out how to repair even a small part of the damage that changed his life."

~ JUDY WOODRUFF

Traumatic brain injury is the disturbance of normal brain function caused by a blow or jolt to the head or penetration of the skull by a foreign object. According to the Centers for Disease Control and Prevention (CDC), about 1.7 million Americans will sustain a traumatic brain injury every year.

The leading causes of traumatic brain injuries are falls, motor vehicle accidents, violence, sports injuries, and explosive blasts. Children, young adults and older adults aged 75 and more are most at risk of traumatic brain injury.

Direct and Indirect Head Injuries.

Head injuries may be direct and indirect.

(1) Direct injuries are caused by a direct blow to the head.

(2) Indirect injuries are caused by the brain colliding against the interior of the skull.

(3) Coup contrecoup injuries are caused by a direct blow to one side of the skull followed by collision of the brain inside the skull, causing an indirect injury on the opposite side.

Coup contrecoup injuries may cause the individual nerves to twist leading to axonal shearing. At first, this creates significant inflammation, and then over the next few months, these nerves begin to die. This is one of the reasons we see decreased electrical activity in the QEEG brain map of patients who have experienced head injuries and concussion.

Mild traumatic brain injuries are those where the resulting confusion, disorientation or lack of consciousness last 30 minutes or less. They account for 75 percent of traumatic brain injuries.

Moderate traumatic brain injuries cause loss of consciousness or post-traumatic amnesia that lasts more than 30 minutes but less than 24 hours.

Severe traumatic brain injuries cause loss of consciousness or post-traumatic amnesia for 24 hours or more.

A sub-concussive event indicates traumatic brain injury even though a full concussion is not reported. This happens often in football linemen because they ram heads with the opposite linemen during every play. According to a study published in the online medical journal PLOS One, researchers at the Cleveland Clinic found that college football players can experience significant brain damage, even when there is no concussion. More than half of the participants showed signs of brain damage, including an auto-immune response and damage to the blood-brain barrier.[1]

Another study from Scotland's University for Sporting Excellence published in *EBioMedicine* has also detected direct changes in the brain after a group of soccer ball players headed a ball 20 times. Increased inhibition in the brain was detected using a basic neuroscience technique called Transcranial Magnetic Stimulation. Memory test performance was also reduced by 41 to 67 percent, though brain function returned to normal within 24 hours. Although the changes were temporary, they may be significant to brain health because they are repeated. Since large numbers of people play soccer around the world, it is important that they are made aware of potential brain damage and its lasting effect.[2]

Complications of traumatic brain injury[3]

Severe and/or repeated head injuries increase the risk of complications such as:

- **Altered consciousness**
  Mild to moderate changes in a person's state of consciousness and responsiveness.

- **Seizures**
  Some serious injuries may result in recurring seizures, called post-traumatic epilepsy.

- **Infections**
  Skull fractures can enable bacteria to enter the brain and cause infections.

- **Blood vessel damage**
  Several small or large blood vessels in the brain may be damaged leading to bleeding in the brain, blood clots, and strokes.

- **Nerve damage**
  Injuries to the base of the skull can damage nerves that emerge directly from the brain (cranial nerves) leading to paralysis of facial muscles, loss of vision, swallowing problems, etc.

- **Sensory problems**
  These include persistent ringing in the ears, blind spots, double vision, impaired hand-eye coordination and dizziness

- **Intellectual problems**
  Many people who have had a significant brain injury will experience changes in their thinking (cognitive) skills. Traumatic brain injury can result in problems with many skills, including memory, learning, concentration, problem-solving, and communication.

- **Behavioral changes**
  People who've experienced brain injury often experience difficulty with self-control, verbal or physical outbursts, and risky behavior.

- **Emotional changes**
  Emotional changes such as anxiety, depression, mood swings, anger or insomnia.

- **Degenerative brain diseases**
  A traumatic brain injury may increase the risk of diseases such as Alzheimer's disease, Parkinson's disease, and Dementia pugilistica.

- **Endocrine Changes**
  30% of patients who have had a TBI develop some type of endocrine imbalance, with the majority of these being thyroid related.

Even a moderate traumatic brain injury is associated with two times the risk of developing Alzheimer's and other dementias. Severe TBI increases that risk by 4.5 times. Individuals who have experienced repeated TBIs are at a higher risk of dementia, cognitive impairment, and neurodegenerative disease.

Some of these conditions, such as Chronic Traumatic Encephalopathy (CTE), are associated with repeated blows to the head. Currently, there is no test to determine if someone has CTE. The only known way to prevent it is to avoid repeated head injuries.

The risk of traumatic brain injury can be reduced by wearing seatbelts, avoiding repeated blows to the head in contact sports, wearing helmets during bicycling, and ensuring a well-lit living environment.

One of the best ways to determine where the damage has taken place in the brain from a TBI is the use of a QEEG brain map. The brain map gives a comparison of the overall magnitude of the individual's brain waves to the normative data base. Any decreased electrical activity around the areas affected by the TBI will most often show up as blue or dark blue which is 1 and 2 standard deviation low. This decrease can be caused by axonal shearing which leads to cell death and thus a lower amount of electrical activity.

References

1. Marchi N, et al. (2013) Consequences of Repeated Blood-Brain Barrier Disruption in Football Players. PLoS ONE 8(3): e56805. doi:10.1371/journal.pone.0056805

2. Di Virgilio, Thomas G., et al. (2016.) Evidence for Acute Electrophysiological and Cognitive Changes Following Routine Soccer Heading. EBioMedicine, 13, 66-71

3. Mayo Clinic. (2014, May 15) Traumatic Head Injury Complications. Retrieved from http://www.mayoclinic.org/diseases-conditions/traumatic-brain-injury/basics/complications/con-20029302

CHAPTER 4

Impact of Aging on the Brain

"Anyone who stops learning is old, whether at twenty or eighty. Anyone who keeps learning stays young."

~ HENRY FORD

The study of aging is more important today than ever because of the increase in life expectancy. According to a 2015 United Nations report on world population aging, the number of people aged 60 and older worldwide will double in the next 35 years. The life expectancy of the average American is nearly 80 years. Though old age brings wisdom and maturity, it also leads to the deterioration of many cognitive abilities such as memory and focus. Despite these improvements in life expectancy, Alzheimer's disease and other neurodegenerative conditions have reached epidemic levels.[1]

The Changing Brain in Healthy Aging

In the past few decades, we have learned much about changes in the brain during healthy aging.

1. As a person gets older, changes occur in all parts of the body, including the brain:
2. Shrinkage of the brain, especially the prefrontal cortex and the hippocampus. Both of these areas are crucial for complex mental activities such as learning, memory, planning, etc.
3. Decrease in communication between neurons because white matter (myelin-covered axons) is damaged or lost.
4. Decrease in the blood flow to the brain because of narrowing of blood vessels and less growth of new capillaries.
5. Development of plaques and tangles within and around neurons.
6. Increased damage of the brain cells by free radicals.
7. Increased inflammation within the brain.[2]

Effects of aging on mental function in healthy older people

Some seniors may notice a slight decline in their ability to remember names and learn new things. Their ability to perform complex tasks of attention, learning, and memory may also be affected. However, the ability of healthy seniors is often similar to those of young adults if given enough time to perform the task. And they may perform better in some areas such as vocabulary and verbal knowledge.

Also, additional brain regions may be activated in older adults during cognitive tasks, such as taking a memory test. Therefore, it is possible that decline in mental abilities is not an inevitable result of aging. There is growing evidence of neuroplasticity in older adults, which may depend on overall health, lifestyle, mental attitude, environment, and genetics.

Another factor in the preservation of a healthy brain in old age is **cognitive reserve**. Cognitive reserve is the brain's ability to function effectively even when some function is disrupted and depends on genetics, education, occupation, lifestyle, leisure activities and other life experiences. It provides the ability to adapt to change and damage that occurs during aging.

Therefore, a person's cognitive reserve as well as genetics, environment, and life experiences may result in normal cognitive function in old age. Whereas another person, with different cognitive reserve, genetics, environment, and life experiences, may be afflicted by a disease process that will ultimately lead to dementia.[2]

Activities that promote brain health in old age

The activities that preserve healthy brain aging also benefit overall health.

They include:

1. A healthy diet that includes plenty of vegetables, fruits, and good fats
2. Regular exercise and physical activity

3. Control of risk factors for chronic diseases such as heart disease and diabetes (blood sugar, blood cholesterol, blood pressure, smoking, and body weight)
4. Maintaining close social ties with family, friends, and community and
5. Intellectually stimulating activities[2]

ACTIVE Study May Provide Clues to Help Older Adults Stay Mentally Sharp

In 2006, the NIA and the National Institute of Nursing Research funded the Advanced Cognitive Training for Independent and Vital Elderly (ACTIVE) study. This study was the first randomized controlled trial to demonstrate long-lasting, positive effects of brief cognitive training in older adults.

The ACTIVE study tested 2,802 healthy adults age 65 and older who were living independently. Participants took part in up to ten computer-based training sessions that targeted specific cognitive abilities such as memory, reasoning, and speed of response to prompts on a computer screen. The investigators tested the participants at the beginning of the study, after the initial training and booster sessions, and once a year for five more years. They found that the improvements from the training counteracted the expected decline in cognitive performance among older people without dementia over 7 to 14 years.

The training also had a positive effect on the everyday lives of the participants. After five years, those who received training reported less difficulty than the control group in tasks such as preparing meals, managing money, and doing housework. However, these results were statistically significant for only the group that had the reasoning training.[2]

References

1. United Nations Department of Economic and Social Affairs, Population Division. (2015.) *World Population Ageing 2015*. Report ST/ESA/SER.A/390. Retrieved from http://www.un.org/en/development/desa/population/publications/pdf/ageing/WPA2015_Report.pdf

2. National Institute on Aging, National Institutes of Health. (2015, January 22.) The Changing Brain in Healthy Aging. Retrieved from https://www.nia.nih.gov/alzheimers/publication/part-1-basics-healthy-brain/changing-brain-healthy-aging

CHAPTER 5

Blood Sugar and the Brain

"I was determined to share my positive approach and not let diabetes stand in the way of enjoying my life."

~PAULA DEEN, CELEBRITY CHEF

Glucose is the main source of energy for every cell in the body. However, the brain uses one-half of all the sugar energy in the body because its nerve cells require the most energy.

Brain functions such as thinking, learning, and memory, are adversely affected if there isn't enough glucose in the brain. Also, hypoglycemia (low glucose levels in the blood) can lead to impaired brain function.

The impact of glucose on the brain is more complicated in diabetes. In type 1 diabetes, the immune system destroys the insulin-producing cells in the pancreas. In type 2 diabetes, dietary and other environmental factors may cause resistance to insulin.

High blood glucose levels can affect the brain's connectivity and cause the brain to shrink. More importantly, it can lead to small-vessel disease, which reduces blood flow in the brain leading to cognitive problems, and eventually, the development of vascular dementia.

In a 2009 study published in *Diabetes Care*, researchers studied people with uncontrolled type 2 diabetes and other risks for cardiovascular disease and found a link between high blood sugar and disturbances in thinking and memory.[1]

Blood sugar and brain function

Higher HbA1c levels worsen brain functions like thinking and memory. The main reason may be damage to small arteries in the brain, leading to mini-strokes and death of brain tissue. The result is a gradual loss of mental function. Another reason is the disruption of the communication pathways within the brain by high blood sugar levels and insulin resistance. Finally, diabetes-related inflammation may result in the development of amyloid plaques in the brain, which is characteristic of Alzheimer's disease.

The danger of low blood glucose

Very low blood sugar (hypoglycemia) can lead to seizures or loss of consciousness in extreme cases. In milder cases, the hypoglycemia will cause slowed cognitive processing, emotional upset, brain fog, and other symptoms of brain fatigue.

The term "hangry" gets applied often to people who become hypoglycemic and become emotionally upset when they get hungry. This can have a profound impact on thinking and memory and can even be life-threatening if not corrected immediately. Hypoglycemia is particularly dangerous in older adults who use insulin or antidiabetic pills.

HbA1c

HbA1c refers to glycated hemoglobin. It reflects the average concentration of glucose in the blood in the last two to three months. For people with diabetes, higher HbA1c levels are linked to a greater risk of diabetes-related complications. HbA1c levels are categorized as follows:

- **normal:** below 5.7%
- **prediabetes:** 5.7%–6.4%
- **diabetes:** 6.5% or above

In 2005 a study was published in the Journal of Neurology where the researchers performed brain scans on the participants and then again one year later. After evaluating the amount of degeneration in the brains, the researchers divided the participants into four categories based on who lost the most amount of brain. A statistical analysis was then performed by the researchers and they determined that HbA1c was the most consistent marker in each of the four categories. Participants with HbA1c even in the 5.3-5.5 range were associated with a 50% greater amount of brain loss than 5.2 and below.

Effect of aging on diabetes and the brain

In the past, the main goal of treating people with diabetes was minimizing complications such as heart disease, kidney failure, blindness, and gangrene of the lower limbs. However, because of more effective treatment strategies, people with diabetes are living longer. As a result, they have to deal with age-related problems such as a decline in brain function and dementia. It is not clear whether these problems are the natural consequences of old age or whether diabetes itself hastens the aging process. Research is being done to establish the underlying mechanisms of neurodegeneration in diabetes.

Is Alzheimer's disease type 3 diabetes?

According to studies carried out at Warren Alpert Medical School at Brown University, there is a much higher percentage likelihood of people that have diabetes to develop diabetes. Basically, if someone with diabetes lives long enough, they will eventually develop Alzheimer's. Therefore, the researchers concluded that Alzheimer's disease represents a form of diabetes that selectively involves the brain and has features that overlap with both type 1 and type 2 diabetes mellitus. So it can be accurately named as type 3 diabetes.[2]

Limiting sugar is crucial to protecting brain health

The average American diet is heavy in sugars and grains. Regularly consuming excessive sugar can lead to insulin resistance and increase your risk of dementia and Alzheimer's disease. It may also increase your brain's craving mechanism, resulting in excessive hunger and subsequent consumption of additional calories, leading to a downward spiral.

References

1. Harvard Mahoney Neuroscience Institute. (n.d.) Sugar and the Brain. Retrieved from http://neuro.hms.harvard.edu/harvard-mahoney-neuroscience-institute/brain-newsletter/and-brain-series/sugar-and-brain

2. de la Monte S.M., Wands J.R. (2008.) Alzheimer's disease is type 3 diabetes—evidence reviewed. J Diabetes Sci Technol, 2, 6, 1101–1113. Retrieved from https://www.ncbi.nlm.nih.gov/pmc/articles/PMC2769828/

CHAPTER 6

Chronic Stress and PTSD

"To wish to be well is a part of becoming well."

~ SENECA

Stress is defined as an uncomfortable emotional experience accompanied by predictable biochemical, physiological and behavioral changes.[1]

Stress can be beneficial when it is short-term and provides the motivation and energy in situations like exams or work deadlines (eustress). However, prolonged stress can adversely affect the heart, brain, gut, blood circulation, immunity, and other functions (distress). Chronic stress can lead to anxiety, sleep disturbances, high blood pressure, high blood sugar, fatigue, muscle pain, obesity, and depression.

Chronic stress leads to prolonged high levels of the stress hormone, cortisol, which triggers many changes in the brain.

Stress affects memory and emotions

Studies show that when you are stressed, there is reduced activity in the hippocampus, which is associated with memories, there is increased activity in the amygdala, which is associated with emotions. Importantly, some of these changes persist even ten days after the cessation of stress.[2]

Stress increases anxiety and fear

Stress increases the size, activity and neural connections in the amygdala. This leads to more anxiety and a vicious cycle of even more stress.[3]

Stress reduces the production of new brain cells

Cortisol halts the production of Brain-Derived Neurotrophic Factor (BDNF), resulting in fewer new brain cells being formed.[4]

Stress reduces serotonin and dopamine leading to depression

Chronic stress reduces levels of neurotransmitters such as serotonin and dopamine, which can make one more prone to depression and addictions. Serotonin plays an important role in mood, learning, appetite control, and sleep. Its deficiency can lead to depression, anxiety, alcoholism, and ADHD. Dopamine plays a role in the pleasure-reward system. Too little dopamine can cause lethargy, lack of motivation, and depression.[5]

Chronic stress shrinks your brain

Stress can measurably shrink your brain, especially the prefrontal cortex, which controls decision-making, working memory, and control of impulsive behavior and the hippocampus, which affects learning, memory, emotional regulation memory and shutting off the stress response after a stressful event is over. Also, there is reduction in gray matter and increase in white matter.[6]

Stress affects the blood-brain barrier

The blood-brain barrier is a filter that protects your brain from harmful substances such as microbes, toxins, chemicals, and heavy metals. Stress makes the blood-brain barrier more permeable, which is called a leaky brain. Having a leaky blood-brain barrier increases the risk of infections, cancers, auto-immunity, and brain damage.[7]

Chronic stress increases your risk of dementia and Alzheimer's disease.

Chronic stress and elevated cortisol contributes to dementia in older adults and hastens its progression.[8]

Stress causes brain cells to commit suicide

Stress leads to premature aging of cells. When a cell divides, it passes on the genetic material to the next cell via chromosomes. Telomeres are protective endcaps on our chromosomes. Every time a cell divides, the telomeres get a little shorter. When telomeres reach a critically shortened length, they signal the cell to stop dividing and the cell dies soon after. Shortened telomeres lead to atrophy of brain cells and longer telomere length leads to the production of new brain cells. The length of telomeres may be a better predictor of risk for age-related diseases like Alzheimer's, heart disease, diabetes, and cancer than conventional diagnostic tools.[9]

Chronic stress contributes to brain inflammation and depression.

Special immune cells called microglia protect the brain and spinal cord from infections and toxins. Unfortunately, chronic stress can activate microglial cells, which produce cytokines and result in inflammation in the brain. This theory is called the cytokine model of depression. Cytokine production is linked to depression, anxiety, memory loss, as well as schizophrenia, Parkinson's, and Alzheimer's disease.[10]

Post-traumatic Stress Disorder (PTSD)

Post-traumatic Stress Disorder is a mental health problem that can develop after experiencing or witnessing traumatic events like war, natural disasters, car accidents, death or injury of a loved one, and physical or sexual assaults. People who continue to have upsetting memories, sleep disturbances or other problems for more than a few weeks or months may have PTSD. Of people who have had trauma, about 1 in 10 men and 2 in 10 women will develop PTSD.[11]

Each person experiences PTSD symptoms in their own way but they may not be exactly the same for everyone. There are four types of PTSD symptoms:

1. Reliving the event
2. Avoiding things that remind you of the event
3. Having more negative thoughts and feelings than before
4. Feeling on edge

People with PTSD may also act in unhealthy ways like smoking, driving aggressively or abusing alcohol and drugs.

PTSD Screen

If you think you might have PTSD, answer the questions in the screening tool below:

1. Have you ever experienced any unusual traumatic event? For example, a serious accident or fire, physical or sexual assault or abuse, earthquake or flood, war, seeing someone killed or seriously injured, or a loved one die through homicide or suicide.

If yes, in the past month, have you:

- Had nightmares about the event(s) or thought about the event(s) when you didn't want to?
- Tried hard not to think about the event(s) or went out of your way to avoid situations that reminded you of the event(s)?
- Been constantly on guard, watchful, or easily startled?

- Felt numb or detached from people, activities, or your surroundings?
- Felt guilty or unable to stop blaming yourself or others for the event(s) or any problems the event(s) may have caused?

If you answered "yes" to three or more of these questions, talk to a mental health care provider to learn more about PTSD and PTSD treatment. Answering "yes" to 3 or more questions does not mean you have PTSD. Only a mental health care provider can tell you for sure.[11]

Reasons to get treatment for PTSD

After treatment, most people feel they have a better quality of life. Getting treatment can help keep PTSD from causing problems in your relationships, your career, or your education — so you can live the way you want to.

Treatment for PTSD[11]

Talk Therapy such as

- Prolonged Exposure Therapy
- Cognitive Processing Therapy
- Eye Movement Desensitization and Reprocessing
- Stress Inoculation Training

PTSD Support groups

Medications such as **SSRIs** (selective serotonin reuptake inhibitors) and **SNRIs** (selective norepinephrine reuptake inhibitors)

Brain Mapping and Neurofeedback

Neurofeedback trains the brain to produce a calm state as well as regulate stress response. Also, the specific areas of the brain affected by PTSD can be targeted. Frequently, the first sign of improvement is that a client's sleep improves. Then other symptoms begin to improve. After sufficient training, someone with PTSD can maintain a calm state on his or her own. When a person has reached this stable state, neurofeedback treatments can be decreased until no further training is needed.

References

1. Baum, A. (1990). «Stress, Intrusive Imagery, and Chronic Distress, *"Health Psychology*, Vol. 6, pp. 653-675.

2. Ghosh S, T. Rao L, and Chattarji S. (2013.) Functional Connectivity from the Amygdala to the Hippocampus Grows Stronger after Stress. Journal of Neuroscience, 33 (17) 7234-7244; DOI: https://doi.org/10.1523/JNEUROSCI.0638-13.2013

3. Pittenger C. and Duman R. S. (2008.) Stress, Depression, and Neuroplasticity: A Convergence of Mechanisms. Neuropsychopharmacology, 33, 88–109. Retrieved from http://www.nature.com/npp/journal/v33/n1/full/1301574a.html

4. Issa G., Wilson C., Terry AV Jr., Pillai A. (2010.) An inverse relationship between cortisol and BDNF levels in schizophrenia: data from human postmortem and

animal studies. Neurobiol Dis.2010 Sep;39(3):327-33. doi: 10.1016/j.nbd.2010.04.017. Retrieved from http://www.ncbi.nlm.nih.gov/pubmed/20451611

5. Tafet G.E., et al. (2001.) Correlation between cortisol level and serotonin uptake in patients with chronic stress and depression. Cogn Affect Behav Neurosci. 2001 Dec;1(4):388-93. Retrieved from https://www.ncbi.nlm.nih.gov/pubmed/12467090

6. J. Bremner D. (2006.) Traumatic stress: effects on the brain. Dialogues Clin Neurosci. 2006 Dec; 8(4): 445–461. PMCID:PMC3181836. Retrieved from https://www.ncbi.nlm.nih.gov/pmc/articles/PMC3181836/

7. Soreq H. and Friedman A. (1996.) Stress may disturb the blood-brain barrier. BMJ 1996;313:1505 Retrieved from http://www.bmj.com/content/313/7071/1505.2

8. Lara V. P. et al. (2013.) High cortisol levels are associated with cognitive impairment no-dementia (CIND) and dementia. Clinica Chimica Acta, 423, 18–22 Retrieved from http://www.sciencedirect.com/science/article/pii/S0009898113001484

9. Epel E, et al. (2009.) Can meditation slow rate of cellular aging? Cognitive stress, mindfulness, and telomeres. Ann N Y Acad Sci., 1172, 34–53. Retrieved from http://www.ncbi.nlm.nih.gov/pmc/articles/PMC3057175/

10. Dobbin JP, Harth M, McCain GA, Martin RA, Cousin K. (1991.) Cytokine production and lymphocyte

transformation during stress. Brain Behav Immun. 1991 Dec;5(4):339-48. Retrieved from http://www.ncbi.nlm.nih.gov/pubmed/1777728

11. National Center for PTSD. (2016.) Understanding PTSD and PTSD Treatment. Retrieved from http://www.ptsd.va.gov/public/understanding_ptsd/booklet.pdf

CHAPTER 7

Autoimmunity in the Brain

"So in the Libyan fable, it is told,
That once an eagle, stricken with a dart,
Said, when he saw the fashion of the shaft,
With our own feathers, not by others' hands,
Are we now smitten."

~ AESCHYLUS

Your immune system is the network of cells and tissues throughout your body that defends you from invasion and infection. Your immune system has two parts:

1. **The innate (or inborn) immune system** activates white blood cells to destroy invaders without using antibodies.
2. **The acquired (or adaptive) immune system** develops as a person grows. It remembers invaders so that it can fight them if they come back. When the immune system is working properly, it activates immune cells and produces antibodies whenever

provoked by foreign invaders. These antibodies then attach themselves to the invaders so that they can be recognized and destroyed.

But sometimes your immune system mistakes your body's own healthy cells as harmful invaders and repeatedly attacks them. This is called an autoimmune disease. ("Autoimmune" means immunity against the self.)[1]

The classic sign of an autoimmune disease is inflammation, which can cause redness, heat, pain, and swelling. How an autoimmune disease affects you depends on what part of the body is targeted. If it affects the joints, as in rheumatoid arthritis, you might have joint pain, stiffness, and loss of function. Many autoimmune diseases can affect numerous parts of the body.

The exact cause of autoimmune diseases is not known. In most cases, a combination of factors is probably at work. For example, you might have a genetic tendency to develop a disease and then, under the right conditions, an outside invader like a virus might trigger it.

The treatment for autoimmunity is to decrease the amount of inflammation and the elevated immune response. From a natural perspective, the way to treat someone with autoimmunity is to address all the different factors that could be driving the immune-inflammatory pathways. These different systems include the blood sugar, adrenals, vitamin D levels, hormones, infections, and many others.

Autoimmune diseases can affect almost any part of the body, including the brain, nerves, heart, muscles, skin, eyes, joints, lungs, kidneys, glands, the digestive tract, and blood vessels.

Autoimmunity in the brain

Auto-antibodies directed against structures in the brain lead to irritation and swelling of brain tissue. If not treated, long-standing inflammation can lead to permanent brain damage and dysfunction.

Guillain-Barré syndrome is a disorder in which the immune system starts to destroy the myelin sheath that surrounds the axons of many peripheral nerves, or even the axons themselves (axons are long, thin extensions of the nerve cells that carry nerve signals). When Guillain-Barré is preceded by a viral or bacterial infection, it is possible that the virus changes the nature of cells in the nervous system so that the immune system treats them as foreign cells. It is also possible that the virus makes the immune system itself less discriminating about what cells it recognizes as its own, allowing some of the immune cells, to attack the myelin.[2]

Multiple Sclerosis is a potentially disabling disease of the brain and spinal cord. The cause of multiple sclerosis is unknown but it is considered an autoimmune disease in which the body's immune system destroys myelin. A combination of genetics and environmental factors may be responsible.

Role of gut microbiome in brain autoimmune disorders

The adaptive immune system may produce auto-antibodies to specific microbes, which may then attack brain cells having similar molecular structure. Interventions that correct the microbiome or decrease autoantibody binding may be effective in different neuropsychiatric conditions mediated by autoimmunity. However, this is an area of ongoing investigation.[3]

Brain injury leading to autoimmune disorders

Repeated hits to the head may lead to neurological disorders later in life, even in the absence of concussion. The cause may be damage to the blood-brain barrier resulting in an autoimmune response. A preliminary study published in *PLOS ONE* journal suggests that the neurodegeneration observed among professional football players could result from an auto-immune response.[4]

The blood-brain barrier is a semi-permeable wall between the brain and bloodstream. It's the only organ in the body to have such a barrier. The barrier holds in proteins and molecules that bathe the brain and protect it from foreign substances. However, blows to the head can damage the blood-brain barrier and allows some proteins from the brain to leak into the bloodstream.

Researchers from the University of Rochester Medical Center and the Cleveland Clinic found that S100B, a protein biomarker for traumatic brain injury, was present in varying degrees in the blood samples of the football players that were tested after every game, even though none of them suffered a concussion. This proves that even sub-concussive hits can affect the blood-brain barrier and perhaps the brain itself.

Results showed that players with the most head hits also had the highest S100B levels and elevated levels of autoimmune antibodies. Players who often remained on the sidelines had significantly lower S100B levels. In addition, the blood samples predicted abnormalities seen in the special brain scans and correlated with observed cognitive changes.

More significantly, the research team also examined what happens after S100B enters the bloodstream from the brain. They discovered that the body views S100B as a foreign invader and begins to form antibodies against it as if it were a harmful microbe. These antibodies then attack the S100B in the bloodstream. Unfortunately, some of these antibodies gain access to the brain through the damaged blood-brain barrier and begin to harm the healthy brain cells that produce the S100B protein. Repeated injury to the blood-brain barrier can lead to repeated auto-immune attacks on the brain cells, which may eventually lead to chronic traumatic encephalopathy.

In multiple sclerosis, a similar breakdown occurs when the body's own immune system damages myelin sheaths around the brain. Other health conditions that harm the blood-brain barrier include sepsis (overwhelming infection), burns, critical illness, or seizures.

Further research may help to understand the genetics and causes of autoimmune disorders in the brain and result in improvement in diagnosing and treating these diseases.

References

1. NIH. NIAMS. (2016, March.) Understanding Autoimmune Diseases. Retrieved from https://www.niams.nih.gov/%5C/Health_Info/Autoimmune/default.asp

2. NIH. NINDS. (2011, July.) Guillain-Barré Syndrome Fact Sheet. Retrieved from https://www.ninds.nih.gov/Disorders/Patient-Caregiver-Education/Fact-Sheets/Guillain-Barr%C3%A9-Syndrome-Fact-Sheet#3139_1

3. Hornig M. (2013.) The role of microbes and autoimmunity in the pathogenesis of neuropsychiatric illness. Curr Opin Rheumatol. 2013 Jul;25(4):488-795. doi: 10.1097/BOR.0b013e32836208de. Retrieved from https://www.ncbi.nlm.nih.gov/pubmed/23656715/

4. Marchi N., et al. (2013.) Consequences of Repeated Blood-Brain Barrier Disruption in Football Players. PLOS ONE. Retrieved from http://journals.plos.org/plosone/article?id=10.1371/journal.pone.0056805

CHAPTER 8

Microbiome

"I am vast. I contain multitudes."

~ WALT WHITMAN

"All disease begins in the gut."

~ HIPPOCRATES

The term microbiome refers to all microorganisms and their genetic material in the body. Microbiota refers to populations of microorganisms present in the body's various ecosystems (for example, the gut microbiota and skin microbiota). The number of microorganisms in the gut is ten times greater than the number of human cells. These microorganisms also contain 150 times more genes than the human genome (all our genes).

Before birth, we do not have any microbes. We acquire our microbiomes from the environment after birth. As we grow up, our microbiomes also change. Within a few years, billions of microbes inhabit most parts of our bodies.

Microbiomes vary with age, gender, climate, diet, hygiene, and occupation. However, there are some similarities. For example, some species of bacteria are found only in the gut, others only on the teeth, and so on. Our microbiomes continue to change in response to illness, fever, injury, stress, changes in diet and antibiotics. Puberty, pregnancy, and menopause can cause big changes in the skin and vaginal microbiomes. After age 65, there is a decrease in the number of microbiome species.

Though many microbes may gain access to the human body, only those that can best adapt to the environment can survive. Similarly, changing an ecosystem can affect the microbiome. For example, changing the diet can influence the microbes in the gut. Excess sugar and processed food may lead to the multiplication of destructive microbes. Taking a prescription antibiotic can kill not just the harmful bacteria, but also the helpful microbes.

Microbiome and disease

Some diseases can disrupt our microbiomes. On the other hand, disturbing our microbiome can cause disease. For example, antibiotics can disturb our microbiome and cause antibiotic-associated diarrhea because they kill not only disease-causing bacteria but also the friendly bacteria that keep us healthy. The loss of these friendly bacteria can allow other types of harmful bacteria to multiply, leading to opportunistic infection. For example, Clostridium difficile can multiply and produce toxins that result in fever, nausea, and diarrhea. Our new understanding may lead to more effective treatments that destroy only the harmful microbes and nurture the helpful ones.[1]

Antibiotic resistance

When an antibiotic is used to treat a bacterial infection, usually all the bacteria are killed. Sometimes, however, a microbe may survive, reproduce, and create more antibiotic-resistant bacteria. Therefore when antibiotics are used incorrectly or too often, it can lead to creation and multiplication of resistant bacteria. Then, doctors are forced to use stronger antibiotics that have more side effects to kill resistant bacteria.

To prevent antibiotic resistance, doctors should prescribe antibiotics only when they are necessary. Also, if you have been prescribed an antibiotic, take the correct dose and complete the full course even if you feel better. We need to use antibiotics responsibly to minimize the spread of antibiotic resistance.[2]

Benefits of microbiomes

Humans and microbes depend on one another: we provide microbes with resources, and they provide functions necessary for our health. Though a few microbes cause disease, most are benign or beneficial and will even support the host immune system and fight off diseases. Many microbes are essential for good health. For example, some microbes coat your inner and outer body surfaces and provide a biological shield against harmful microbes. Many microbes play an important role in the production of vitamins like Vitamin B12 and break down food that you can't digest on your own. They also boost immunity, reduce inflammation, and the risk of cancer.

The gut microbiome plays a major role in the two-way communication between the gut and the brain. For example, formation of short-chain fatty acids by carbohydrate fermentation can affect brain functions. The vagus nerve may transmit hormonal, neuronal, and bacterial changes in the bowel to the brain. The gut microbiome produces neuroactive substances such as serotonin and GABA and BDNF (brain-derived neurotrophic factor).[3]

The gut microbiome may have an influence on mood. Regulation of the gut microbiota using diet, probiotics, and fecal microbiota transplantation may help to prevent and treat depression. In the next ten years, microorganisms may be used for the treatment of psychiatric disorders (psychomicrobiotics).[4]

ADD and microbiome

Many studies have been performed in recent years looking at the effect the microbiome has on people's attention and focus. One of the studies done at Ohio State University evaluated the microbiome of participants between 18 months and 4 years of age. They assayed the fecal matter of participants to determine the variety of strains of good bacteria and the total volume. They also had parents and teachers fill out questionnaires assessing the overall focus and hyperactivity of the children. The researchers found there was a direct correlation between the two. Children who had more total microbiome and a broader variety had better attention and behavior, while those that had the least amount and variety had more issues.

Ways to improve gut microbiome

Probiotics are beneficial bacteria that exist in your gut and in fermented or "living" foods such as yogurt, sauerkraut, kombucha, kefir, kimchi, fermented vegetables, and probiotic supplements.

Prebiotics like inulin are non-digestible fiber found mostly in plants and other carbohydrates that promote the growth of beneficial bacteria. They are present in onions, asparagus, leeks, bananas, garlic, chicory roots, dandelion greens, and prebiotic supplements.

Activated charcoal binds to bacterial toxins and inhibits their absorption. It is used to reduce diarrhea, indigestion and bloating symptoms in various diseases.

Fecal microbiota transplantation using feces from a spouse or a relative is used to treat infection by Clostridium difficile and inflammatory bowel diseases like ulcerative colitis and Crohn's disease.

References

1. Khanna S, Tosh PK. (2014.) A clinician's primer on the role of the microbiome in human health and disease. Mayo Clin Proc.;89:107–114. doi: 10.1016/j.mayocp.2013.10.011. Retrieved from https://www.ncbi.nlm.nih.gov/pubmed/24388028

2. Hawkey, P.M. (1998.) The origins and molecular basis of antibiotic resistance. British Medical Journal, 317(7159), 657-660.

3. Alper Evrensel and Mehmet Emin Ceylan (2015.) The Gut-Brain Axis: The Missing Link in Depression. Clin Psychopharmacol Neurosci. 2015 Dec; 13(3): 239–244. Retrieved from https://www.ncbi.nlm.nih.gov/pmc/articles/PMC4662178/

4. Genetic Science Learning Center. (2014, August 15.) The Human Microbiome. Retrieved from http://learn.genetics.utah.edu/content/microbiome/

CHAPTER 9

Medications

*"If I'd known I was going to live so long,
I'd have taken better care of myself."*

~ LEON ELDRED

A variety of medications can affect the brain. Alcohol abuse may cause dementia or dementia-like syndromes. Recreational drugs, as well as over-the-counter and prescription medications, may cause a range of cognitive impairments from confusion to delirium, and may even mimic dementia. Polypharmacy (use of more than five drugs), which is common among older adults, increases the risk of adverse interactions that may interfere with cognition.[1]

Anticholinergic medications

Medications with anticholinergic effect block the action of the neurotransmitter acetylcholine, often as a side effect. Acetylcholine is a biochemical with a wide range of functions including memory and cognitive function. So long-term use of these medications has been linked to cognitive impairment and memory loss. Doctors are not aware of all of the medications their patients take or the anticholinergic properties of the ones they prescribe. Unfortunately, older patients, who tend to take more medicines, are also more vulnerable to their effects.

Symptoms caused by anticholinergic medications:

- cognitive impairment
- confusion
- delirium
- hallucinations
- rapid heart rate
- dry mouth
- constipation
- inability to urinate
- decreased sweating and fever
- skin flushing
- difficulty with vision (dilatation of pupils)

One study of more than 13,000 British men and women aged 65 or older for two years, found that those taking more than one anticholinergic drug had lower cognitive function and death rate was 68 percent higher than those who were not taking any such drugs.[2]

The list of drugs with anticholinergic properties includes Paxil (antidepressant), Benadryl (cough syrup) and allergy medications. Many other drugs such as digoxin (heart drug), warfarin (blood thinner), codeine (opiate painkiller) and prednisone (steroid) are mild anticholinergics. Many over-the-counter drugs, including antihistamines and Tylenol PM, have anticholinergic effects.

Every year, ask your doctor to review the collective anticholinergic effect of all your medications, including non-prescription and alternative medicines. Do not stop medications on your own without medical supervision.

You can also do your own research by using the Anticholinergic Cognitive Burden Scale.[2]

Developed by the Aging Brain Program of the IU Center for Aging Research, it lists drugs with definite and possible anticholinergic effects and suggests alternatives.

Alcohol use and cognitive impairment among older adults

Alcohol is the most commonly used recreational drug in older adults. Moderate to high alcohol consumption is one of the risk factors for the development of dementia before age 65. Heavy alcohol consumption is neurotoxic and causes shrinkage of total cortical and subcortical volume. On the other hand, prolonged abstinence leads to gradual improvement of cognitive ability.

Marijuana

Use of marijuana is associated with acute neuropsychological effects such as disturbance of attention, short-term memory, and executive functioning, which may continue for years after abstinence.

Narcotic painkillers such as morphine and codeine

They are commonly prescribed for pain relief but their use can result in deficit in attention, concentration, recall, executive functions and other cognitive functions. Also, they are highly addictive.

Polypharmacy

Daily use of more than five drugs increases the risk of adverse drug reactions. In the U.S., polypharmacy is found in 40% of people older than 65 years.

References

1. Rogers J., Wiese B. S., and Rabheru K. (2008.) The Older Brain on Drugs: Substances That May Cause Cognitive Impairment. Geriatrics and Aging. 2008;11(5):284-289. Retrieved from http://www.medscape.com/viewarticle/579841

2. Fox C, et al. (2011.) Anticholinergic medication use and cognitive impairment in the older population: the medical research council cognitive function and ageing study. J Am Geriatr Soc. 2011 Aug;59(8):1477-83. Retrieved from http://www.ncbi.nlm.nih.gov/pubmed/21707557

3. The Aging Brain Program of the IU Center for Aging Research. (n.d.) The Anticholinergic Cognitive Burden Scale. Retrieved from http://lbdtools.com/files/antichol_burden_scale.pdf

CHAPTER 10

Effect of Sleep on the Brain

"Sleep is the death of each day's life."

~ WILLIAM SHAKESPEARE

Getting a high quality and restorative sleep every night should be a priority because sleep is as important as good nutrition, hydration, and exercise. The brain *needs* quality sleep to function properly. Lack of quality sleep during the night, may result waking up the next day feeling, tired, groggy, and cranky. Sleep is necessary to feel alert, be productive and creative and for optimal body functioning.

During sleep, your brain repairs the neurons (neuroplasticity) and the connections between them (synaptic plasticity). It also consolidates memories from the brain. Finally, it clears toxins and eliminates waste products while sleeping, which reduces the risk of dementia and Alzheimer's disease.[1]

Importance of daylight light exposure

People who get enough natural sunlight during the day get better sleep at night. However, we do not get enough natural light during the day and use too much artificial light at night. This affects our natural circadian rhythms, hormones, and immunity.

Blue light emitted from digital devices such as computers, TVs, and cell phones is beneficial during the day as it boosts your attention and improves your mood. However, at night, exposure to blue light interferes with sleep.

Sleep deprivation health effects

Sleep deprivation, even for a few hours at night, impacts cognition (thinking), mood, memory and learning. People with insomnia are twice as likely to develop dementia. Chronic sleep deprivation can lead to depression, weight gain, increased risk of diabetes and cancer and increased risk of accidents.[2]

Sleep deprivation can affect brain function in the following ways:

- increasing amyloid-β concentrations
- interfering with memory formation
- disrupting circadian rhythm and melatonin production
- causing lack of oxygen by breathing disorders while sleeping
- causing depression

Obstructive sleep apnea

This is a sleep-related breathing disorder during which breathing may decrease or even stop temporarily. Obstructive sleep apnea may not be noticed because these changes happen during sleep. However, your sleeping partner may complain of loud snoring at night. Depending on the severity, you may feel drowsy and tired during the day, which results in low productivity, road accidents, and workplace accidents. Also, due to reduced oxygen supply, you are at greater risk from brain damage (micro-infarcts) and heart disease.

According to the American Academy of Sleep Medicine, 12 percent of American adults suffer from obstructive sleep apnea. Fortunately, it is treatable. After treatment, affected individuals benefit from better sleep quality, greater productivity and a 40 percent reduction in absence from work after treatment.[3]

Nine ways to improve your sleep quality

You can reduce the health risks associated with sleep deprivation by sleeping eight hours each night and improving the quality of sleep.

1. Prepare for sleep

Do not do work or use computers or cells phones or watch television in bed. Reduce interruptions from family, friends, and pets.

2. Establish a pre-bedtime routine

Stop working and watching TV at least one hour before bed so that you get a chance to relax before falling asleep. A warm bath, reading a good book or meditation will help you to get a good night's sleep. Lavender essential oil diffused in the bed room can help the quality of sleep.

3. Maintain a consistent sleep schedule

Go to bed and wake up at the same time even on the weekends so that your body and brain get used to it.

4. Get plenty of exposure to daylight sunlight

Exposure to daylight in the morning signals to your body that it's time to wake up and stops production of melatonin. A morning walk outdoors will not only give you the benefit of exercise but also boost production of vitamin D.

5. Reduce lights after dark

Dim the lights and turn off electronic devices after sunset. Normally, your brain starts secreting melatonin between 9 p.m. and 10 p.m., which can be inhibited by bright lights and electronic devices. Use low-wattage lights with yellow, orange or red light after dark. Dimmer switches are easy to install and allow the lights to become lower as the night progresses.

6. Block blue light at night

Install blue light-blocking software like f.lux (http://justgetflux.com) on your computer and smartphone. This free software automatically reduces blue light after sunset. Another solution is to use amber-colored glasses that block blue light. For example, the S1933X Uvex model (https://www.amazon.com/dp/B000USRG90) costs $9 and eliminates almost all blue light. Once you wear it, it doesn't matter which light sources you use at night.

7. Exercise daily

Exercise improves the quantity and quality of sleep. However, the body also releases cortisol during exercise, which may reduce the secretion of melatonin. So exercise at least three hours before bed.

8. Keep your room cool and dark

During sleep, the body's temperature drops to its lowest level. The optimal temperature for good sleep is between 60 and 68 degrees Fahrenheit.

9. Check your mattress and pillow

Make sure your mattress and pillows are comfortable as well as supportive; they should not be too soft or too hard.[4]

References

1. Kang JE, et al. (2009.) Amyloid-beta dynamics are regulated by orexin and the sleep-wake cycle. Science. 2009 Nov 13;326(5955):1005-7. doi: 10.1126/science.1180962. Retrieved from https://www.ncbi.nlm.nih.gov/pmc/articles/PMC2789838/

2. Dr. Mercola. (2014, March 27.) How Dangerous Is Sleep Deprivation, Really? Retrieved from http://articles.mercola.com/sites/articles/archive/2014/03/27/sleep-deprivation-risks.aspx

3. The American Academy of Sleep Medicine. (2016, August 8.) Economic burden of undiagnosed sleep apnea in U.S. is nearly $150B per year. Retrieved from http://www.aasmnet.org/articles.aspx?id=6426

4. Dr. Mercola. (2016, September 8.) What Lack of Sleep Does to Your Brain Retrieved from http://articles.mercola.com/sites/articles/archive/2016/09/08/sleep-deprivation-brain-health.aspx

CHAPTER 11

Mold Exposure

"An oppressive odor of decay now mingled with the stench of mold and seemed to clutch at the very breath in their lungs."

~ KAORU KURIMOTO, THE LEOPARD MASK

Mold is fungi that grow in the form of multicellular thread-like structures called hyphae. (Fungi that exist as single cells are called yeasts.) Some molds like penicillin are useful but others can cause food spoilage or disease.

Mold growth requires moisture, which can be from washing, cooking, condensation, leaks from plumbing, and so on. Toxic molds such as Aspergillus, Stachybotrys, and Fusarium growing in your home, school, or workplace can cause serious health problems. Everyone is potentially at risk from toxic mold exposure.

Mycotoxins

Molds release spores, many of which may contain mycotoxins. More than 200 types of mycotoxins have been identified. Because of the weed killers *RoundUp* and *glyphosate* and antifungal paint in construction, only the strongest molds survive and they release more toxins in response to the hostile environment.[1]

These toxins can be absorbed through your intestinal lining, airways, and skin and can cause many health problems. These toxins cause progressive damage and can contribute to cancers, respiratory problems, autoimmune conditions, and neurotoxicity.

The main reason why mycotoxins are so dangerous is they can cross directly into your brain after they are inhaled. Neurotoxicity due to mold exposure can give rise to any of the following symptoms: headaches, insomnia, anxiety, depression, tremors, brain fog, disorientation, irritability, involuntary muscle movements, and short or long-term memory loss.

Mycotoxins can break down myelin (covering of nerves) leading to neurodegenerative diseases like Alzheimer's disease, Parkinson's disease, and multiple sclerosis.[2]

Prevention and management of problems caused by mold exposure

Proper medical help

The symptoms of mold sensitivity and exposure can be easily mistaken for other conditions like fibromyalgia or chronic fatigue. Therefore, it's important to consult a doctor who specializes in the treatment of mold exposure.

Proper Diet

Choose an anti-inflammatory diet that is low in sugar and contains high-quality fats and proteins. Avoid gluten, yeast, wheat, corn, grain, barley, peanuts, cottonseed, chocolate, mushrooms, and grain-fed meat and dairy, which may have high mycotoxin levels. Unfiltered tap water, unfiltered alcoholic beverages (especially beer and wine) and commonly available coffee may also contain high mold mycotoxin levels. Use a water filter for drinking and bathing as chlorine in the water will amplify the negative effects that mycotoxins have on the body.

Supplements

Take high-quality supplements that promote detoxification in your body such as S-acetyl glutathione, resveratrol, pine bark extract, and turmeric.

How to prevent and manage toxic mold in your home

Mold in your home, school, or workplace can pose a number of serious health problems. Here are some ways to prevent or minimize the risk of exposure to mold:

- Avoid living or working in any building that has been damaged by water.
- Have the pipes in your home professionally inspected for leaks.
- Have your home and office inspected for an intact moisture barrier in the walls.

- Ensure you have proper ventilation because toxic mold flourishes in moist environments that lack proper airflow.
- Before renting or buying real estate, perform a gravity mold test (www.immunolytics.com). This type of test will help determine the specific strains and amount of mold present in the area.
- If testing reveals the presence of toxic mold in your environment, get it cleaned by a remediation specialist.
- Most commercial mold products are also highly toxic. Make sure that the products being used to deal with mold are not doing more damage than good. CitriSafe (www.citrisafe.com) is a company with citrus-based products that will help remove mold and be safe for you as well.

References

1. Dave Asprey. (2016.) Why Mycotoxins Are Kryptonite (And How to Hack Them). Retrieved from https://blog.bulletproof.com/why-mycotoxins-are-kryptonite/

2. Monnet-Tschudi F, Zurich MG, Sorg O, Matthieu JM, Honegger P, Schilter B. (1999.) The naturally occurring food mycotoxin fumonisin B1 impairs myelin formation in aggregating brain cell culture. Neurotoxicology, 20(1):41-8. PMID: 10091857. Retrieved from https://www.ncbi.nlm.nih.gov/pubmed/10091857

Resources

Dave Asprey. (2016.) Free Mold Risk Awareness Report. Retrieved from http://blog.bulletproof.com/wp-content/uploads/2015/06/Moldy-Mold-Awareness-Report.pdf

Dave Asprey. (2016.) Online mold archive: Research & References. Retrieved from http://www.betterbabybook.com/research/

National Treatment Centers for Environmental Disease. (2016.) Mold Exposure and the Human Brain. Retrieved from http://ntced.org/mold-exposure-human-brain/#

CHAPTER 12

Neurofeedback

"To get the body in tone, get the mind in tune."

~ ZACHARY T. BERCOVITZ

*"All sorts of bodily diseases are
produced by half-used minds."*

~ GEORGE BERNARD SHAW

Neurofeedback is a safe, non-invasive, drug-free method that targets irregular brainwaves using a computer. Proper brainwave function improves attention, focus, memory, and sleep. Neurofeedback has been clinically proven to improve most neurological conditions such ADHD, learning disabilities, depression and chronic pain.

Neurofeedback does not directly target conditions and symptoms; instead, it corrects irregular brainwaves and modifies timing patterns in the brain. This is achieved over multiple sessions, as the brain is re-trained into normal patterns. The result is an improvement in brain regulation, which can impact a variety of symptoms.

The brain produces four primary types of brain waves:

1. **Beta** brain waves are dominant when you are awake.
2. **Alpha** brain waves are seen during relaxed states when your eyes are closed but you are not asleep.
3. **Theta** brain waves are present briefly during the periods before you fall asleep and before you fully wake up.
4. **Delta** brain waves are primarily active when you are asleep.

All of these brain waves are equally important to your health. Neurological disorders can be attributed to irregularity in specific brain waves.

Your brain can be compared to a musical quartet. When all four musicians are playing synchronously, they produce harmonious music. But if even one musician is out of tune, the result can be disastrous. Brainwaves operate in much the same way, working together to keep your mind and body in sync and running smoothly. But if any of the brainwaves are irregular, it affects the functioning of the brain. Many common conditions like anxiety and depression can occur when brainwaves are running too fast or too slow. Neurofeedback trains the brain to regulate its brainwaves, which results in better overall health.

People who suffer from neurological symptoms have irregular brainwaves. For example, a person with ADD has **slower beta** brainwaves, which are responsible for attention and focus. They also have **faster theta** brainwaves, which can lead to daydreaming. A head injury may cause **excessive frontal theta** or **delta**, the slower waves, when you are supposed to be awake and alert. By retraining these abnormal patterns in the affected areas, symptoms can be improved or eliminated. Neurofeedback can improve alertness, attention, emotional regulation, behavior, cognitive function, and mental flexibility.

Neurofeedback is commonly used as an adjunct or alternative treatment to medication and behavior management. It can:

- Improve **depression** symptoms by speeding up Alpha brainwaves
- Improve **autism** symptoms by speeding up Beta brainwaves
- Improve **sleep disorders** by slowing Delta brainwaves
- Improve **memory** by speeding up Theta brainwaves
- Increase **attention and focus** for children with attention deficit disorders
- Reduce **cravings** in persons with **addiction** and
- Reduce **anxiety and stress** by slowing down Beta brainwaves

Neurofeedback sessions involve relaxing for 30 minutes while you watch a movie or listen to music or audio books of your choice. Electrodes are attached to your scalp, which monitor your brainwaves during the session. When irregular patterns are detected, a response is triggered from the software that pauses or dims the video or music. This change is not annoying but it automatically causes you to refocus, which will restore your brainwaves back to the normal range. At that time the movie or music will resume normally. This process is called **operant conditioning**. With repetition of this process over multiple sessions, you can retrain your brain to stay within healthy ranges on its own. At that time, no further neurofeedback sessions are needed.

Neurofeedback does not require any medication. All it requires is your attention for 30 minutes per session. You can continue your medication during neurofeedback. Usually, the same dosage seems to have a stronger effect on a more efficient brain. As you progress, your physician might suggest that you slowly reduce or eliminate certain medications related to the condition being treated with neurofeedback. However, since every patient is unique, the decision to reduce medication will depend on your physician. This is because neurofeedback restores normal brainwave function. Over time, you may be able to eliminate all medications completely.

Neurofeedback is safe because it is non-invasive, requires no drugs and does not produce any radiation like a CT scan. Each session usually lasts 30 minutes. The number of sessions needed depends on the individual and the particular condition. Usually, 20 to 40 neurofeedback sessions may be required to improve or even eliminate most neurological symptoms. However, positive changes are seen after just the first few sessions.

Results vary from person to person. Some may feel the difference within a couple of sessions, while others may take more sessions to see any noticeable results. It's important to be patient. The practitioner will be able to show you the graph results of each session, which will provide a visual reference of improvement.

If neurofeedback is not done properly, problems may arise. That is to be expected from a system that can produce such positive changes. It all comes down to training and proper use. Fortunately, each session is designed to create small changes in brainwave activity, meaning that problems can be spotted and corrected before they become bigger. Our clinic has extensive training on this equipment and can change protocols as needed if negative effects are seen.

Neurofeedback has been in use since the 1960s. Initially, Dr. Joe Kamiya discovered that people could learn to alter their brain activity by using a simple reward system. His partner, Dr. Sterman, discovered that he could train cats to control their epileptic seizures through a similar method. He moved on to train humans to control their epilepsy.

Neurofeedback has evolved over the years from laboratory research to a system that can be administered in an office setting. Advances in computer technology in the past ten years have made it possible for doctors to easily administer neurofeedback in their clinics.

Five decades of positive case studies have proved its effectiveness in improving brain health. Long-term follow up has been done on many patients over the years. For example, Dr. Joel Lubar at the University of Tennessee has followed ADD clients who have sustained their improvement from neurofeedback for 10-20 years. Thousands of studies have been published to date. The American Academy of Pediatrics has given a Level One recommendation to neurofeedback as a tool for ADD/ADHD. This is the same recommendation as medications and talk therapy.

The following conditions are clinically responsive to neurofeedback:

1. ADD / ADHD
2. Addiction
3. Anger Management
4. Anxiety
5. Autism
6. Bipolar Disorder
7. Brain Injury
8. Chronic Pain / Fatigue
9. Concussion / Brain Injury
10. Depression
11. Dyslexia
12. Epilepsy
13. Fibromyalgia
14. Insomnia and sleep disorders
15. Lyme Disease
16. Memory Loss
17. Alzheimer's disease
18. Migraines
19. OCD
20. Stress and PTSD
21. Schizophrenia
22. Seizures
23. Stroke,
24. Tourette's syndrome and more!

References and Resources

Dr. Ben Galyardt. (2016.) Neurofeedback. Retrieved from http://www.neurofeedbackfortcollins.com

1. Dr. Ben Galyardt. (2016.) Conditions Clinically Responsive To Neurofeedback. Retrieved from http://www.neurofeedbackfortcollins.com

2. Dr. Ben Galyardt. (2016.) Research on Neurofeedback. Retrieved from http://www.neurofeedbackfortcollins.com/research/

3. Dr. Ben Galyardt. (2016.) Common Questions about Neurofeedback. Retrieved from http://www.neurofeedbackfortcollins.com/#faqs

4. Dr. Ben Galyardt. (2016.) Videos from Patients and Doctors. Retrieved from http://www.neurofeedbackfortcollins.com/videos/

CHAPTER 13

QEEG Brain Map

*"I wish my brain had a map to tell
me where my heart should go."*

~ UNKNOWN

Electroencephalography (EEG) is a non-invasive test that measures brainwave patterns using surface electrodes. Quantitative EEG (qEEG) is the analysis of the digitized EEG using a computer. In qEEG, the brainwave measurements are mapped onto a picture of the head or brain and represented as different colors. Therefore, it is also called brain map.

The data from the brain map is then compared with benchmark standards of normal brain function to determine any problems. Though it does not identify specific conditions, it shows a map of problem areas in the brain that the doctor can use to identify potential conditions. Brain mapping can also be used to evaluate and track the changes in brain function due to neurofeedback or medication.

The FDA has approved brain mapping software for clinical use by qualified medical or clinical professionals for the diagnosis of ADD/ADHD.[1]

A brain map is the most accurate tool available for identifying irregular brainwaves. It also generates a set of protocols that can correct specific brainwave irregularities using neurofeedback.

Brain Mapping is painless, safe, accurate and non-invasive. It's the best way to analyze brainwaves and collect customized data about brain function for each individual.

The Five Types Of Brainwaves[2]

All humans display five different types of electrical patterns or "brain waves" across the cortex. Each brain wave has a purpose and helps serve us in optimal mental functioning.

Though the EEG displays all five types of brain waves, one type of brain wave will be dominant depending on the state of the brain at the time of the EEG.

1. Beta Waves

Beta brainwaves are dominant when we are alert, attentive, solving problems, making decisions, and engaged in focused mental activity.

- Optimal beta activity results in enhanced focus, memory, and problem-solving skills.
- Too little beta activity may indicate ADHD, daydreaming, depression, and poor cognition.
- Too much beta activity uses up a huge amount of energy and may indicate high arousal, inability to relax, anxiety, and stress.
- Coffee, energy drinks, various stimulants can increase beta activity.

2. Alpha Waves

Alpha brainwaves are dominant in meditative states and tranquil thinking states. Alpha is the resting state for the brain and bridges the gap between our conscious thinking and subconscious mind. Alpha waves enhance relaxation, mental coordination, learning, and mind-body integration. When we become stressed, a phenomenon called "alpha blocking" may occur, which involves the beta waves "blocking" the production of alpha waves.

- Optimal alpha activity indicates relaxation
- Too little alpha activity indicates anxiety, high stress, insomnia, and OCD
- Too much alpha activity indicates daydreaming and inability to focus
- Alcohol, marijuana, relaxants, some antidepressants can increase alpha activity.

3. Theta Waves

Theta brainwaves are dominant in sleep, deep meditation, and as we wake or drift off to sleep. Theta waves are connected to the experience of deep emotions. Theta can enhance intuition, creativity, and deep relaxation.

- Optimal theta activity indicates creativity, relaxation, intuition, and emotional connection,
- Too little theta activity indicates stress, anxiety, and poor awareness of emotions.
- Too much theta activity indicates depression, hyperactivity, ADHD, inattentiveness, and extreme impulsivity.
- Alcohol, sedatives and LSD can increase theta activity.

4. Delta Waves

Delta brainwaves are responsible for sleep, rest and recharging.

Delta brainwaves are the slowest brain waves in human beings. They are associated with the deepest levels of meditation and dreamless sleep. Delta waves enhance healing and rejuvenation especially during deep sleep.

- Optimal delta activity improves immunity, natural healing, and restorative sleep
- Too little delta activity indicates poor sleep and failure to heal the body and brain
- Too much delta activity can indicate concussion, learning problems, inability to think, and severe ADHD
- Depressants and sleep increase delta waves.

5. Gamma Waves

Gamma brainwaves are the fastest brain waves and are associated with simultaneous processing of information from different areas of the brain. So they enhance learning, memory, and information processing. Gamma is highly active in states such as love, altruism, and expanded consciousness.

- Optimal gamma activity indicates improved learning, perception, information processing and REM sleep
- Too much gamma activity indicates stress, anxiety, and high arousal.

- Too little gamma activity indicates ADHD, depression, and learning disabilities
- Meditation increases gamma waves

Conclusion

Brain mapping can detect brain waves in all areas of the brain and identify the areas where the brain is not functioning properly. It takes the guesswork out of the assessment process and provides an accurate road map for improving your health and well being.

The Brain Map Report

This comprehensive report of findings shows the problem areas of the brain and how to improve them with neurofeedback. The data is easy to read.

Samples pages from the brain map are below.

MAGNITUDE

| Delta | Theta | Alpha | Beta |

○ Very High
● High
● Normal
○ Low
◐ Very Llow

DOMINANT FREQUENCY

| Delta | Theta | Alpha | Beta |

○ Very High
● High
● Normal
○ Low
◐ Very Llow

ASYMMETRY

| Delta | Theta | Alpha | Beta |

○ Very High
● High
● Normal
○ Low
◐ Very Llow

This page shows an analysis of each lobe of the brain (frontal, parietal, central, temporal and occipital) for each type of brain wave: Delta, Theta, Alpha, and Beta. Green indicates a normal level, red is elevated and yellow is extreme.

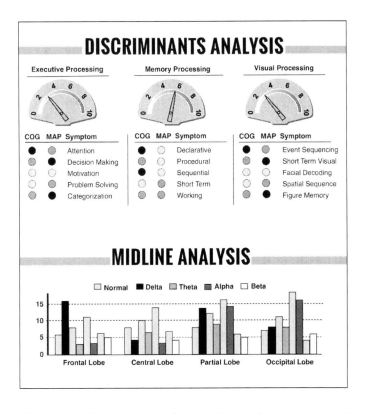

The **Discriminants Analysis page** (above) shows a visual meter for the major functions of the brain, such as the cognitive, emotional, memory processing, executive functions, and more.

The **Emotional and Cognitive Analysis** compares the results of your self-assessment against the results of the brain map and helps identify problem areas within the brain. Red indicates a strong potential match; green indicates no match.

EMOTIONAL ANALYSIS

- Physiological Anxiety
- Obsessional Thinking
- Hyper Vigilance
- Worry
- Hyper-arousal
- Anger
- Emotionally Impulsive
- Self-Deprecation
- Excessive Rationalization
- Victim Mentality
- Hyperactive Attention
- Dislike of Novelty
- Over Control of Emotion
- Emotional Rumination
- Irritability
- Socially Cavalier
- Socially Inappropriate
- Passive Aggressiveness
- Excessive Self-Concern
- Lack of Self-Awareness

COGNITIVE ANALYSIS

EXECUTIVE PROCESSING
- Attention
- Categorization
- Decision Making
- Motivation
- Problem Solving

VERBAL PROCESSING
- Dialogue Organization
- Short Term Verbal
- Tone Sequencing
- Verbal Sequencing

MEMORY PROCESSING
- Declarative
- Episodic
- Procedural
- Short Term (Digit Span
- Working

VISUAL PROCESSING
- Event Sequencing
- Facial Deciding & Recognition
- Figure Memory
- Short Term Visual Memory

The Midline Analysis is a visual reference of your brainwaves compared to normal ones. Gray bars are normal levels; color bars are from your brain map.

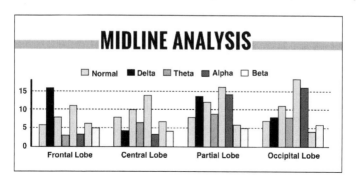

89

References

1. U.S. Food and Drug Administration. (2017, February 6.) Product classification. Retrieved from http://www.accessdata.fda.gov/scripts/cdrh/cfdocs/cfpcd/classification.cfm?ID=3470 (Normalizing Quantitative Electroencephalograph Software.)

2. Dr. Ben Galyardt. (2016.) The Brain Map. Retrieved from http://www.neurofeedbackfortcollins.com

CHAPTER 14

Oxygen Therapy

*"Your memory needs oxygen as fuel,
so why not feed it often?"*

~ TONY BUZAN

*"Even the laziest person will fight
for oxygen when drowning."*

~ J. R. RIM

Oxygen therapy improves brain function and quality of life by inhalation of 100% oxygen in a total body chamber, where atmospheric pressure is increased and controlled.

Hyperbaric oxygen is a simple, painless, drug-free, and non-invasive treatment. During hyperbaric oxygen therapy, oxygen is dissolved into all of the body's fluids and reaches all areas, including those where the blood circulation is blocked or reduced. So, extra oxygen can reach damaged tissues and boost the body's healing process naturally and with minimal side effects. Therefore, it can be used for treatment of a wide range of conditions.

Hyperbaric oxygen is used to treat all conditions that will benefit from increased tissue oxygenation such as:

1. decompression sickness (Bends)
2. carbon monoxide poisoning
3. gas gangrene
4. air embolism
5. crush injury
6. diabetic wounds
7. severe blood loss and anemia
8. intracranial abscess, etc.

It is also used to treat:

1. traumatic brain injury
2. stroke
3. sports injuries
4. autism
5. cerebral palsy
6. Lyme disease
7. migraine
8. multiple sclerosis and other neurodegenerative disorders

Live oxygen therapy increases the oxygen carried in the blood, which helps to heal damaged capillary walls, prevents plasma leakage and reduces swelling. This restores blood flow to the areas damaged by trauma or stroke and improves healing and neurogenesis.

A study on the effect of hyperbaric oxygen on mild traumatic brain injury reported significant improvement in cognitive function and quality of life as well as elevated brain activity. The study was carried out on 56 patients with mild traumatic brain injury and prolonged post-concussion syndrome, 1 to 5 years after injury. There was significant improvement in cognitive function and quality of life after 40 HBOT sessions of 60 minutes each, with 100% oxygen at 1.5 ATA (atmospheres absolute).[1]

Another study published in PLOS One on 74 patients who suffered stroke 6–36 months earlier and had at least one motor dysfunction reported significant improvements such as renewed use of language, enhanced sensation, and reversal of paralysis of all patients. The results indicate that hyperbaric oxygen therapy can lead to significant neurological improvements in post stroke patients even at chronic late stages.[2]

Oxygen Multi-Step Therapy

It was developed by Professor von Ardenne in the late 1960s and combines oxygen therapy, drugs that facilitate intracellular oxygen turnover, and physical exercise. Oxygen Multi-Step Therapy is now called Exercise with Oxygen Therapy (EWOT). The heart of this therapy is the breathing of pure oxygen while exercising, which dramatically increases the amount of oxygen absorbed into the blood circulation and tissue fluids.

There are three technologies that can deliver different levels of oxygen to the body:

1. **Hyperbaric oxygen therapy:** It delivers about 20 liters of oxygen per minute and requires about 20 to 60 hours of therapy.

2. **Exercise with oxygen therapy (EWOT):** It delivers about 5 to 10 liters of oxygen per minute and requires about 36 hours of therapy.

3. **Live Oxygen (LiveO2):** It delivers more than 50 liters of oxygen per minute and requires 15 minutes or less of therapy. So Live Oxygen is more effective, convenient and cheaper than hyperbaric oxygen or other exercise with oxygen therapies.

Live Oxygen

The original Oxygen Multi-Step Therapy consisted of an 18-day, 36-hour program. The LiveO2 system reduces it to only 15 minutes a day and gives the same benefit in the first 15-minute session. What is true for hyperbaric oxygen therapy is exponentially true for Live Oxygen Therapy. Though oxygen bars and hyperbaric chambers have become popular, they do not give the same benefits as the Live Oxygen training system.

Live Oxygen ensures that the maximum amount of oxygen reaches where it is needed the most: to damaged and inflamed tissues. It specifically targets capillary inflammation and restores the blood micro-circulation, boosts blood supply to tissues and allows them to return to normal aerobic metabolism. Live Oxygen starts a healing process where normally there would be none because there is no cellular energy for it.

Live Oxygen Apparatus consists of an oxygen concentrator, a reservoir that stores up enough oxygen for a fifteen-minute session, an oxygen mask, and an exercise bicycle, treadmill or jumper. A graded exercise program along with oxygen begins the transformation process. If you can get on a bicycle or treadmill, you can enjoy a veritable fountain of youth for the cells. Increasing your oxygen levels not only increases your state of well being but also has anti-aging and weight-loss effects.

LiveO2 Adaptive Contrast™

If you're athletic, LiveO2 Adaptive Contrast doubles the performance of LiveO2. LiveO2 AC switches between high oxygen and reduced oxygen. It's easy to breathe with high oxygen and it lets your heart and lungs take it easy. LiveO2 Adaptive Contrast switches you to the equivalent of an elevation of about 14,000 feet. This switch makes your heart and lungs work harder and enables the oxygen to do much more. For athletes, LiveO2 Adaptive Contrast is a training accelerator that gets rid of waste and soreness from their muscles in less than 15 minutes. So they are able to recover from intense training and competition much faster, usually in about one-third the normal time.

Oxygen is vital for every physiological function of the human body. Irrespective of present your level of physical and mental health, you will benefit by flooding your cells with oxygen.

References

1. Boussi-Gross R, Golan H, Fishlev G, Bechor Y, Volkov O, Bergan J, et al. (2013) Hyperbaric Oxygen Therapy Can Improve Post Concussion Syndrome Years after

Mild Traumatic Brain Injury - Randomized Prospective Trial. PLoS ONE 8(11): e79995. doi:10.1371/journal.pone.0079995

2. Efrati S., et al. (2013). Hyperbaric Oxygen Induces Late Neuroplasticity in Post Stroke Patients – Randomized, Prospective Trial. PLoS ONE, 8(1): e53716 doi: 10.1371/journal.pone.0053716

Useful links

Live Oxygen website (http://Liveo2.com)

Harch Hyperbaric Oxygen Therapy website (http://HBOT.com)

CHAPTER 15

Supplements

"A man may esteem himself happy when that which is his food is also his medicine."

~ HENRY DAVID THOREAU

Supplementation is one of the best ways to help the brain rejuvenate. Below is a list of some of the most researched supplements available.

1. S-Acetyl Glutathione

Glutathione is the body's master antioxidant. It is made up of three amino acids: cysteine, glycine and glutamine, and contains a sulfur group, which attaches to the toxins in the body and removes them safely.

Unlike the other antioxidants, glutathione is intracellular and enhances the activity of all the other antioxidants. It removes toxins from our cells and protects us from the damaging effects of radiation, chemicals, and environmental pollutants.

Since glutathione protects all parts of the cell, including the mitochondria, it has a role to play in the prevention and treatment of neurological disorders like Alzheimer's disease, Parkinson's disease, dementia, and multiple sclerosis. Glutathione helps healthy people by boosting their immunity against infectious disease, toxins, pre-cancerous cells and the aging process. In athletes, glutathione improves strength and endurance, and decreases fatigue, muscle pain, and recovery time from injury.

Glutathione deficiency has been linked to:

- Age-related diseases such as Alzheimer's and Parkinson's disease
- Coronary and autoimmune diseases
- Arthritis, asthma, and other inflammatory conditions
- Cancer
- Muscle weakness and fatigue[2]

Three ways to increase your glutathione levels:

1. **Food:** Eat foods that are high in sulfur like garlic, onions, broccoli, cabbage, and cauliflower as well as kale and collard greens.
2. **Exercise** directly increases glutathione levels.
3. **Supplements:** Glutathione is available as intramuscular injection, intravenous injection and topical patch. Most oral glutathione preparations supplements do not get absorbed. However, it is postulated that the acetylation of glutathione combined with leading-edge nanotechnology may permit molecules to pass through the cellular barriers more easily allowing your body to reap the positive effects of this life-enhancing natural medicine.

2. Resveratrol

Resveratrol is found in red wine, chocolate, peanuts, berries, grapes seeds and grape skins. It protects cardiac health and prevents many age related illnesses. Resveratrol's effects on diabetes, cancer, aging, and neurological diseases are being studied worldwide.

Resveratrol is a natural polyphenol developed by grapes to combat bacteria and fungi, and to withstand drought, ultraviolet radiation and nutrient deficiencies. In humans, it acts as an antioxidant and lowers the risk of developing chronic diseases.

Cardioprotective effects: Resveratrol inhibits LDL cholesterol oxidation, which can lead to atherosclerosis. It may also increase HDL cholesterol and improve endothelial function.

Chemopreventive effects: Resveratrol reduces proliferation of human cancer cells and also improves immunity and anti-inflammatory activity.

Anti-aging effects: Resveratrol can reduce the deleterious effects of the aging process.

Neuroprotective effects: Because of its ability to cross the blood-brain barrier, resveratrol protects nerve cells from damage and prevents the buildup of plaque that can lead to Alzheimer's disease.

Autoimmunity Effects: Chronic inflammation is a known risk factor for diabetes, heart disease, rheumatoid arthritis, and cognitive diseases. Resveratrol helps to inhibit major inflammatory pathways because of its powerful anti-inflammatory properties.[3]

Placing a resveratrol lozenge under the tongue enables it to be directly absorbed into the blood stream. This enables a lower dose to be used because it minimizes its breakdown in the digestive tract or liver.

3. Huperzine A

Huperzine A is a substance derived from a plant called Chinese club moss. It causes an increase in the levels of acetylcholine, which is a neurotransmitter needed for communication by nerves in the brain, muscles, etc. So Huperzine A improves memory, concentration, mental clarity, and learning ability.[4]

Huperzine A is used in the treatment of Alzheimer's disease and age-related dementia. It is also used for treating a muscular disorder called myasthenia gravis.

4. Omega-3 fatty acids

Omega-3 fatty acids are essential polyunsaturated fatty acids. The use of omega-3 fatty acids improve mental function and reduce the severity of Alzheimer's disease, ADHD, dyslexia, brain atrophy, and cognitive decline. Sources include fish, flax seeds, walnuts, spinach, etc.

The three main types of omega-3 fatty acids are:

a. **Alpha-lipoic acid (ALA)** is mostly found in many plant foods, including kale, spinach, purslane, soybeans, walnuts, chia seeds, flax seeds, and hemp seeds. ALA is not biologically active and needs to be converted into EPA or DHA. Unfortunately, this conversion process is inefficient in humans.

b. **Eicosapentaenoic acid (EPA)** is mostly found in seafood, including fatty fish and algae. It fights inflammation in the body and can reduce depression.

c. **Docosahexaenoic Acid (DHA)** is found in high amounts in seafood, including fatty fish and algae, and grass-fed animal products. It is important for brain development in children and optimum brain function in adults. It may also help protect against cancer, heart disease, and inflammation.

5. Vitamin D

Vitamin D is a steroid hormone, obtained either from sun exposure or supplementation, along with some foods. About half or more of the general population is at risk of vitamin D deficiency. Vitamin D protects against infections, chronic diseases, and cancers. Several studies have confirmed that vitamin D supplementation can also help alleviate the symptoms of depression.[5]

6. Vitamin K2

Vitamin K is a fat-soluble vitamin. "K" comes from the German word "*koagulation*" because it has a role in blood clot formation.

There are two types of vitamin K:

- **K1 (phylloquinone)** functions mainly in the liver. Its natural sources are green leafy vegetables and some plant oils. It is needed for blood coagulation.
- **K2 (menaquinones)** is found in the brain. Its dietary sources are fermented dairy products (kefir), fermented soybean products (natto) as well as grass-fed beef and liver. It boosts overall cognitive function prevents damage to neurons by free radicals and makes bones stronger. It also protects again inflammation and cancer. Eating vitamin K-rich foods sharpens memory and helps to prevent or delay dementia in older adults.

Vitamin K works best when taken with other fat-soluble vitamins. Choose vitamin K supplements that include K1 and K2 with both MK-4 and MK-7. Always take vitamin K and other fat-soluble vitamins after meals containing fats. Consult your doctor first if you take blood thinners like warfarin. The recommended daily dose is 2000 mcg/day.

7. Turmeric (curcumin)

Turmeric is used not only as a spice but also as a natural medicine in traditional Chinese and Indian medicine for thousands of years. Its active ingredient, curcumin, acts as a powerful antioxidant in the brain. It increases the production of BDNF (Brain-Derived Neurotrophic Factor) and boosts memory, reduces fatigue and enhances mood. Studies have shown that turmeric acts as an anti-aging agent and decreases symptoms of Alzheimer's disease.[7]

References

1. Dr. Ben Galyardt. (2015, May 29.) Essential Vitamins and Minerals for Managing ADHD. Retrieved from https://www.linkedin.com/pulse/6-essential-vitamins-minerals-managing-adhd-dr-ben-galyardt

2. Dr. Theresa Ramsey (2010.) Glutathione for Life! The Most Underutilized Supplement! Retrieved from http://www.drramsey.com/glutathione-for-life-the-most-underutilized-supplement/

3. Dr. Mercola. (2015, September 28.) Resveratrol May Offer Protection Against Alzheimer's. Retrieved from http://articles.mercola.com/sites/articles/archive/2015/09/28/resveratrol-alzheimers-disease.aspx

4. Ben Greenfield. (2012.) 12 Mental Performance Hacks: A Cheat Sheet For Boosting Your Brain Power. Retrieved from https://bengreenfieldfitness.com/2012/01/12-mental-performance-hacks/

5. Dr. Mercola. (2016.) Health Conditions in Which Vitamin D Plays an Important Role. Retrieved from http://articles.mercola.com/sites/articles/archive/2016/01/06/vitamin-d-role-in-health-conditions.aspx

6. Dave Asprey. (2016.) Build A Stronger Brain With Vitamin K. Retrieved from https://blog.bulletproof.com/build-a-stronger-brain-with-vitamin-k/

7. Mishra S. and Palanivelu K. (2008.) The effect of curcumin (turmeric) on Alzheimer's disease: An overview. Ann Indian Acad Neurol. 2008 Jan-Mar; 11(1): 13–19. doi: 10.4103/0972-2327.40220. Retrieved from http://www.ncbi.nlm.nih.gov/pmc/articles/PMC2781139/

CHAPTER 16

Food for the Brain

*"Let food be your medicine,
and medicine your food."*

~ HIPPOCRATES

"Food is our most important drug."

~ BARRY SEARS

One of the best ways to improve brain function is to include brain-boosting foods to your diet. Most of these foods help to improve not only your brain but also your overall health because they contain essential nutrients.

Here are 15 of the best brain-boosting foods that can be eaten every day:

1. Walnuts

Walnuts resemble little brains, which indicate they are good for the brain! They contain omega-3 fatty acids, which are important for memory and concentration. Walnuts also contain antioxidants such as vitamin E and polyphenols, which protect brain cells from damage by environmental and dietary toxins.[1]

2. Almonds

Almonds are an important source of essential nutrients including folate, tocopherol, polyphenols and unsaturated fatty acids. Almonds may prevent or delay the onset of age-associated cognitive dysfunction and improve memory.

3. Coconut Oil

Coconut oil has unique health benefits, especially as a brain-boosting food. Unlike other saturated fats, coconut doesn't have long-chain fatty acids that can raise triglycerides and LDL cholesterol. Instead, it contains **medium-chain fatty acids,** which are easily absorbed. Medium-chain fatty acids can be converted to ketones, which are helpful in memory loss and symptoms of Alzheimer's disease.[2] For best results, use organic unrefined coconut oil.

4. Flaxseed Oil

Flaxseed oil prevents oxidative stress in the brain and improves memory and cognitive function. Flaxseed oil can get spoiled when exposed to heat and light, so it must be stored in dark bottles and refrigerated.

5. Chia Seeds

Chia seeds contain high levels of antioxidants that protect brain cells. Chia seed is a rich source of omega-3 fatty acids in the form of ALA (alpha-linolenic acid). Chia seeds absorb as much as 12 times more water than their weight and forms a gel-like substance. When consumed, this gel can help people feel full and prevent spikes in blood sugar after meals.

6. Pumpkin Seeds

Pumpkin seeds are a rich source of zinc. Low levels of zinc may have a role to play in learning disabilities, schizophrenia, and other brain disorders like Wilson's disease. Pumpkin seeds are usually called *pepitas*, the Spanish word for pumpkin seed. Raw pumpkin seeds contain more nutrients than roasted seeds. You can add pumpkin seeds to your salads, curry recipes, and salad dressings.

7. Leafy Greens

Leafy greens such as spinach, kale, watercress, mustard greens, romaine, and Swiss chard protect against neurodegenerative diseases like Alzheimer's disease. This is because leafy greens are high in vitamin E and other essential nutrients.[3]

8. Sauerkraut

Sauerkraut (fermented cabbage) contains high levels of dietary fiber and vitamin A, vitamin C, vitamin K, and B vitamins. It is also a good source of proteins and minerals such as calcium, iron, sodium, manganese, magnesium, and copper. Sauerkraut contains many helpful micro-organisms that help restore your balance of healthy gut bacteria (microbiome).

9. Eggplant

Eggplant (aubergine) is an edible egg-shaped, purple fruit of a species of nightshade. It is called brinjal in Southeast Asia and South Africa. Eggplant contains an anthocyanin called nasunin, which is a neuroprotective antioxidant. Anthocyanin has been shown to reduce neurodegeneration in Parkinson's Disease by improving mitochondrial function.[4]

10. Hemp

Though hemp and marijuana are both from the cannabis plant, hemp is not psychoactive. Hemp contains amino acids, vitamin E, and omega-3 fatty acids, which may help to prevent diseases like Parkinson's and Alzheimer's disease.[5]

11. Quinoa

Quinoa is rich in antioxidant vitamins like vitamin E, which protects and improves brain function. Also, quinoa is the only plant food that contains all nine essential amino acids. These amino acids form high-quality proteins, which are required to make neurotransmitters such as dopamine, serotonin, and norepinephrine.

12. Apples

Apples contain flavonoids such as quercetin and vitamin C, which prevent oxidative damage of brain cells. An apple a day keeps brain degeneration away!

13. Berries

Berries are low-glycemic fruit and recommended in diabetes. All berries such as raspberries, blackberries, strawberries, blueberries, acai berries, cranberries, and goji berries prevent and decrease neurodegeneration because of their high antioxidant content. Berries may also improve neuron communication and memory.

14. Organic Eggs

The yolk in organic eggs contains choline, which is essential for brain development and memory. Lifelong improvement in memory was seen in two-week-old rats that were fed choline supplements.[6]

15. Fish liver oil

Fish liver oil contain alpha-3 omega fatty acids, an essential nutrient for brain health that improves cognitive function and protects brain cell membranes.[7] Omega-3 fatty acids may reduce the severity of ADHD, dyslexia, Alzheimer's disease, brain atrophy and cognitive decline. Fish oil also contains vitamin A and Vitamin D, which helps to reduce inflammation and boost immunity.

References:

1. Vinson JA, Cai Y. (2012.) Nuts, especially walnuts, have both antioxidant quantity and efficacy and exhibit significant potential health benefits. Food Funct. 2012 Feb;3(2):134-40. doi: 10.1039/c2fo10152a. Retrieved from http://www.ncbi.nlm.nih.gov/pubmed/22187094

2. Fernando WM, et al. (2015.) The role of dietary coconut for the prevention and treatment of Alzheimer's disease: potential mechanisms of action. Br J Nutr. 2015 Jul 14;114(1):1-14. doi: 10.1017/S0007114515001452. Retrieved from http://www.ncbi.nlm.nih.gov/pubmed/25997382

3. Gómez-Pinilla F. (2008.) Brain foods: the effects of nutrients on brain function. Nat Rev Neurosci. 2008 Jul;9(7):568-78. doi: 10.1038/nrn2421. Retrieved from http://www.ncbi.nlm.nih.gov/pmc/articles/PMC2805706/

4. Strathearn KE, et al. (2014.) Neuroprotective effects of anthocyanin- and proanthocyanidin-rich extracts in cellular models of Parkinson's disease. Brain Res. 2014 Mar 25;1555:60-77. doi: 10.1016/j.brainres.2014.01.047. Retrieved from http://www.ncbi.nlm.nih.gov/pubmed/24502982

5. Lee MJ, et al. (2011.) The effects of hempseed meal intake and linoleic acid on Drosophila models of neurodegenerative diseases and hypercholesterolemia. Mol Cells. 2011 Apr;31(4):337-42. doi: 10.1007/s10059-011-0042-6. Retrieved from http://www.ncbi.nlm.nih.gov/pmc/articles/PMC3933972/

6. Nutritional importance of choline for brain development. Zeisel SH. (2004.) Nutritional importance of choline for brain development. J Am Coll Nutr. 2004 Dec;23(6 Suppl):621S-626S. Retrieved from http://www.ncbi.nlm.nih.gov/pubmed/15640516

7. Kidd PM. (2007.) Omega-3 DHA and EPA for cognition, behavior, and mood: clinical findings and structural-functional synergies with cell membrane phospholipids. Altern Med Rev. 2007 Sep;12(3):207-27. Retrieved from http://www.ncbi.nlm.nih.gov/pubmed/18072818

CHAPTER 17

BDNF in the brain

*"I fast for greater physical
and mental efficiency."*

~ PLATO

Brain-derived neurotrophic factor (BDNF) is a protein that plays a vital role in stimulating new brain cell formation (neurogenesis) and maintaining the health of existing brain cells. Its production is mediated via a gene located on chromosome 11. BDNF helps to protect the brain from the destructive effects of chronic stress.[1]

Eight Ways to increase BDNF Levels (Brain-Derived Neurotrophic Factor)[2]

BDNF (Brain-Derived Neurotrophic Factor) influences brain function as well as the peripheral nervous system. Low levels of BDNF have been linked to poor brain development, dysfunction of neurotransmitters, obesity, depression, Alzheimer's disease, and even schizophrenia. Therefore, it's vital to maintain optimal levels of BDNF.

Here are some specific ways to increase BDNF levels:

1. Intense Exercise

One of the most effective ways to increase BDNF is intense exercise. The greater the intensity, the greater is the production of BDNF. Also, it is important to exercise regularly. Try to maintain 60% to 75% of your max heart rate for approximately 30 minutes. There are many psychological benefits of exercise on the brain besides just increasing BDNF. However, it may take up to a few months of regular exercise to produce a significant increase in BDNF level.

2. Restriction of calories or intermittent fasting

Caloric restriction or intermittent fasting increases BDNF within the brain, which not only improves brain health but also cardiovascular functioning and control of blood glucose levels. Similar to exercise, elevation of BDNF is seen only after a few months of consistent caloric restriction and intermittent fasting.[3]

3. Healthy nutrition

A diet containing large amounts of refined sugar and saturated fats reduces hippocampal BDNF, neuronal plasticity, and learning. It can take about two months for BDNF levels to increase in response to a healthy diet.[4]

4. Reduction of weight

High body weight and obesity are linked to decreased production of BDNF because those with elevated bodyweight are less likely to fast, restrict calories or do regular intense exercise. Lifestyle changes to reduce weight may not only increase BDNF but also improve mood. For example, increased BDNF levels in those with metabolic syndrome improved depressive symptoms. Women with higher BDNF levels were in better shape and scored higher in cognitive tests of Total Recall and Delayed Recall. BDNF may also play a direct role in childhood obesity. Restricting calories, improving diet and regular exercise may reduce obesity and increase BDNF levels.[5]

5. Exposure to sunlight (Vitamin D)

Sufficient sunlight (and adequate production of Vitamin D) increase BDNF levels. One study demonstrated BDNF levels increased in the spring and summer and decreased in the fall and winter. BDNF levels were also affected by the number of hours of exposure to sunshine. Those who don't get enough sunlight throughout the year have decreased BDNF levels.[6] Low BDNF levels may lead to depression in the fall and winter. Such people may benefit from Vitamin D supplementation.

6. Social engagement

A good way to increase BDNF levels is by improving social relationships and interaction. This can result in long-term brain and behavioral changes. Positive social experiences, right from childhood, may lead to increased brain plasticity in adulthood. This increase in plasticity may be caused by high BDNF levels.

7. Supplements

The following supplements may help to increase BDNF production:

a. **Curcumin**: Curcumin, the active ingredient in turmeric, may promote BDNF production in the hippocampus, especially among those with brain injuries.

b. **Green tea**: Unfractionated green tea polyphenols as well as their active ingredient, epigallocatechin-3-gallate, increase BDNF levels.

c. **Omega-3 fatty acids**: These essential fatty acids are found in fish, seafood, fish liver oil supplements, etc. Docosahexaenoic acid (DHA) is specifically responsible for increasing BDNF levels. In people with brain injuries, supplementation of omega-3 fatty acids helps to restore BDNF back to normal levels.

d. **Resveratrol** is used in the prevention and treatment of neurodegenerative diseases. Its neuroprotective effect may be because it mediates increase in BDNF levels.

Low serum BDNF was associated with lower cognitive test scores and mild cognitive impairment. The above actions can help to restore BDNF levels back to normal. However, it can take a few months to restore deficient BDNF levels to normal.

References

1. Exercise and time-dependent benefits to learning and memory. Berchtold NC, Castello N, Cotman CW. (2010.) Exercise and time-dependent benefits to learning and memory. Neuroscience. 2010 May 19;167(3):588-97. doi: 10.1016/j.neuroscience.2010.02.050. Retrieved from http://www.ncbi.nlm.nih.gov/pmc/articles/PMC2857396/

2. Mental Health Daily. Mental Health Blog. (2016.) 8 Ways to Increase BDNF Levels (Brain-Derived Neurotrophic Factor). Retrieved from http://mentalhealthdaily.com/2015/03/30/8-ways-to-increase-bdnf-levels-brain-derived-neurotrophic-factor/

3. Mattson MP. (2005.) Energy intake, meal frequency, and health: a neurobiological perspective. Annu Rev Nutr. 2005;25:237-60. Retrieved from http://www.ncbi.nlm.nih.gov/pubmed/16011467

4. Molteni R, et al. (2002.) A high-fat, refined sugar diet reduces hippocampal brain-derived neurotrophic factor, neuronal plasticity, and learning. Neuroscience. 2002;112(4):803-14. Retrieved from http://www.ncbi.nlm.nih.gov/pubmed/12088740

5. Pillai A, et al. (2012.) Plasma BDNF levels vary in relation to body weight in females. PLoS One. 2012;7(7):e39358. doi: 10.1371/journal.pone.0039358. Retrieved from http://www.ncbi.nlm.nih.gov/pubmed/22768299

6. Molendijk ML, et al. Serum BDNF concentrations show strong seasonal variation and correlations with the amount of ambient sunlight. PLoS One. 2012;7(11):e48046. doi: 10.1371/journal.pone.0048046. Retrieved from http://www.ncbi.nlm.nih.gov/pmc/articles/PMC3487856/

CHAPTER 18

Exercise

"A feeble body weakens the mind."

~ JEAN-JACQUES ROUSSEAU

"Exercise is king and nutrition is queen. Together you have a kingdom."

~ JACK LALANNE

"Old minds are like old horses; you must exercise them if you wish to keep them in working order."

~ JOHN ADAMS

The World Health Organization ranks physical inactivity as the fourth biggest preventable killer globally. Regular exercise helps you to lose weight, improves the quality of sleep, increase immunity, lowers your risk of diabetes, heart disease, and cancer, and improves your mental and emotional health. A study published in the New England Journal of Medicine reported that consistent moderate exercise decreased risk of death by 44%.[1]

The two most common kinds of exercise are strength training and aerobic exercise.[2]

STRENGTH TRAINING

It means doing work against resistance using your own body weight, resistance bands, or free weights such as dumbbells and barbells.

Benefits of strength training:

- Improves the strength of your muscles
- Improves muscular movement and coordination by improving your neural drive.
- Increases metabolic rate and thus helps in burning fat and reducing weight.
- Improves insulin sensitivity and thus helps in the prevention and control of diabetes.
- Increases glucose usage as muscle tissue has the only cells in the body that can use glucose without needing insulin to assist with the uptake.
- Reduces anxiety, improves memory and cognition, reduces fatigue, and boost your happiness.
- Increases bone density.
- Increases testosterone and Human Growth Hormone (HGH), leading to muscle growth and fat loss in both men and women.

AEROBIC EXERCISE

It includes any exercise that depends on and improves the capacity of your heart, lungs and blood circulation such as jogging, swimming, biking, and dancing.

Benefits of aerobic exercise:

- improves aerobic capacity by strengthening your lungs.
- increases BDNF (brain-derived neurotrophic factor) resulting in improved learning and memory. BDNF also protects your brain from damage, and promotes the growth of new brain cells (neurogenesis).
- reduces body fat more than resistance training.
- improves mood, possibly by releasing feel-good neurochemicals called endorphins.
- boosts mental flexibility and creativity.

HIGH-INTENSITY INTERVAL TRAINING (HIIT)

HIIT combines strength training and aerobic training and gives the benefits of both. It's a type of interval (anaerobic) training in which short bursts of high-intensity exercise are alternated with gentle recovery periods.[2]

For example, you may run for 30 seconds, then walk for 30 seconds, do squats for 30 seconds, then walk for 30 seconds, and so on. Not only does HIIT give greater benefits than a traditional cardio workout, but it also increases production of HGH (human growth hormone) and helps to delay the degenerative effects of aging.

However, the biggest benefit of HIIT is that it's extremely time-effective. Instead of weight-training or jogging for an hour, you need to do HIIT for only about 15-20 minutes. Also, you don't need equipment and you can do it at home.

During a HIIT workout, we:

1. alternate between intense and mild exercise.
2. alternate between upper and lower body exercises.
3. exercise for a fixed duration using a timer (or our smartphone alarm).
4. slow down or rest more if we become tired, and take care to avoid any injury.

HIIT increases production of Human Growth Hormone (HGH)

We have three types of muscle fibers:

- **Slow muscle fibers** are red muscles that contain abundant oxygen because they are filled with capillaries and mitochondria. They are used during traditional aerobic exercise and strength training.
- **Fast muscle fibers** are also red muscles but are five times faster than slow muscle fibers. These muscles are used during plyometric burst type of exercises (muscles exert maximum force in short intervals of time with the goal of increasing power.) Example: specialized repeated jumping.
- **Super-fast muscle fibers** contain far less blood and less densely packed mitochondria. These muscles are used for anaerobic short burst exercises in HIIT.

Aerobic exercise and strength training engage only your slow muscles. HIIT *engages both fast and super-fast twitch muscle fibers and increases the production of HGH*, also known as the fitness hormone. HGH burns your excess fat, promotes muscle growth, and promotes overall health and longevity.[3]

Sample HIIT workout

Do each exercise for 30-45 seconds followed by active walking for 30-45 seconds.

You can adapt it according to your fitness level, especially if you haven't exercised recently. For example, exercise for a shorter period or exercise less intensely or rest whenever required during the workout.

- **Twists** for 30-45 seconds
- Walk in place for 30-45 seconds
- **Jog in place** for 30-45 seconds
- Walk in place for 30-45 seconds
- **Push-ups** for 30-45 seconds
- Walk in place for 30-45 seconds
- **Bodyweight squats** for 30-45 seconds
- Walk in place for 30-45 seconds
- **Push-ups** for 30-45 seconds
- Walk in place for 30-45 seconds
- **Sit-ups** for 30-45 seconds
- Walk in place for 30-45 seconds
- **Lunges** for 30-45 seconds
- Walk in place for 30-45 seconds

Tabata workout

You can also try a Tabata workout, named after its creator, Dr. Izumi Tabata. Choose any exercise such as push-ups, squats or lunges. Do the exercise intensely for 20 seconds followed by rest for 10 seconds. Repeat eight times.

For example,

1. Do squats for 20 seconds
2. Rest for 10 seconds
3. Repeat the same sequence seven times more (total: 8 times).

So the Tabata workout takes only four minutes but it's an intense workout.

Please consult your doctor before you start any exercise routine.

References

1. Paffenbarger R S Jr., et al. The Association of Changes in Physical-Activity Level and Other Lifestyle Characteristics with Mortality among Men N Engl J Med 1993; 328:538-545February 25, 1993DOI: 10.1056/NEJM199302253280804

2. HIIT: Hack your Muscles, Happiness, and Creativity in One Go Bulletproof Staff. (2017.) HIIT: Hack your Muscles, Happiness, and Creativity in One Go. Retrieved from https://blog.bulletproof.com/hiit-hack-your-muscles-happiness-and-creativity-in-one-go/

3. Dr. Mercola. (2012, November 02.) High-Intensity Interval Training and Intermittent Fasting - A Winning Combo for Fat Reduction and Optimal Fitness. https://blog.bulletproof.com/hiit-hack-your-muscles-happiness-and-creativity-in-one-go/

CHAPTER 19

Functional Neurology

"Functional neurology encompasses all therapeutic interventions which can change the function, and therefore, the structure of the nervous system through neuroplasticity. This may include but is not limited to chiropractic adjustments, exercises, drugs, and/or supplements."

~ DAVID TRASTER DC

What makes functional neurology unique is the use of the latest advances in neuroscience with specific diagnostic and treatment modalities that improve function within all neurological pathways, from sensation to perception, movement to thought and learning."

~ KARLA MEHLENBACHER DC

*My number one priority is the
health and healing of my patients
and Functional Neurology gives me
the best answer to do that."*

~ JASON MCCLOSKEY CSCS, CPT, BSC
(PRESIDENT, PARKER UNIVERSITY
NEUROLOGY CLUB)

Functional neurology is on the cutting edge of health care. Traditionally, neurology tends to look at diseases of the nervous system as black-and-white with one side being optimal neurologic function and the other being neurological disease such as tumors, strokes, degeneration, etc. Functional Neurology is an exciting approach to healthcare because it regards dysfunction of the nervous system as different shades of gray in the nervous system before they become distinct pathologies.[1]

Neurons need fuel and activation in order to thrive and survive. Fuel can be defined as oxygen, glucose and essential nutrients. Activation refers to stimulation of the nervous system, which causes changes in the structure and metabolism of the nerve cell. More recently, Functional Neurology Practitioners are also engaged in eliminating possible negative effects on neurons such as toxins, infectious agents, and immune responses.[1]

The four important factors in functional neurology care are:

1. determining the location of the failure in the nervous system and/or body

2. determining the right stimulation to activate that area

3. determining the health and condition of the failing area, so as to establish how much stimulation would be excessive, and

4. adapting this vital information in order to apply the precise amount of stimulation[1]

The stimulation must be specific to the patient who is being treated. There is bio-individuality in the nervous system, which is as individual as fingerprints. Even those with similar symptoms may require different stimulations at different frequencies and intensities in order to achieve the best success. This cannot be done in a generalized or cookbook type program. For example, you cannot treat every patient with a balance disorder or ADHD with the same treatment protocols.

Generalized treatments run the risk of stimulating an area of the nervous system that is already overexcited or stimulating an area that should be inhibited. Results are maximized when the program of stimulations is tailored to the individual patient's problem and capacity, instead of a one-size-fits-all program where results may be limited or the program may actually be inappropriate. In other words: Different people, different brains, and therefore, different treatments.

It is important to note that the functional neurological examination, though very detailed, is noninvasive and therefore can be performed on different patients without causing any anxiety or discomfort. This is significant especially for practitioners treating children on the autism spectrum because these children tend to have higher anxiety.

The skilled Functional Neurology Practitioner knows that everything from the patient's posture to his tics, faulty eye movements, and alignment are all expressions of what is going on in the patient's nervous system. Subtle though these expressions may be, to the highly skilled Functional Neurologist, these little details mean a lot.

Activation of the nervous system via specific exercises or stimulations to targeted areas of the brain, pathways or circuits can create powerful results in the patient. However, this activation should be carefully monitored; so that the metabolic capacity of the patient's nervous system is not exceeded, which may result in fatigue instead of the intended rehabilitation.

Functional neurology is a field of study that achieves successful results by applying current neuroscience in an office setting. This means that the Functional Neurology Practitioner is taking current neuroscience from the research laboratory and devising ways of applying that research in the office to treat patients. The training begins with neuron theory and progresses to a level that allows the practitioner to evaluate and treat dysfunction of the nervous system. This is done either without or in conjunction with medications.

The following is a list of health conditions people have shown significant improvement with:

1. balance disorders
2. arm / shoulder pain
3. low back pain / sciatica
4. bulging / herniated discs
5. carpal tunnel syndrome
6. dizziness
7. dystonia
8. early Alzheimer's symptoms
9. fibromyalgia
10. restless leg syndrome (RLS)

11. headaches
12. migraines
13. insomnia
14. hip / knee / feet pain
15. tremor disorders
16. MS symptoms
17. neck pain
18. numbness
19. spinal stenosis
20. low immunity[1]

Contemporary health care innovation seems to be gradually distancing itself from the definition of medicine as simply a treatment or manufactured cure. Instead, it's embracing the possibilities of creating conditions for optimal functioning: early prevention, wellness and thriving. The wave of "Functional Neurology" expresses a similar wisdom.

The vision of Functional Neurology has been present for generations; however its momentum as a legitimate medical modality and discipline is more recent. It links and integrates chiropractic knowledge, psychology, conventional medicine, optometry, audiology, and physical and occupational therapies to offer both a form of brain training for outstanding performance and a powerful system of healing for disorders rooted in the nervous system.

A Functional Neurologist differs from a conventional neurologist in his or her basic attitude towards care and medical intervention. A conventional neurologist is led by an understanding of structural pathology and depends on pharmaceutical and surgical initiatives. On the other hand, a Functional Neurologist recognizes the plasticity of the nervous system, its capacity for change, ongoing learning, and marvelous adaptability.

The functional neurologist views the neuron and the nervous system as central to human wellness and expression. So it follows that much of the diagnostic process is based on evaluation of the quality of three basic functions carried out in all neurons. These three functions are:

1. sufficient gas exchange, particularly the exchange of oxygen and carbon dioxide, and its attendant blood flow
2. sufficient nourishment, such as glucose and a series of key cofactors and essential compounds, and

3. sufficient connection and communication between neurons, including inhibition and activation through synaptic activation.

The synaptic activation of a neuron spurs the stimulation of immediate early genes and second messengers within the neuron, which then leads to DNA transcription of appropriate genes and the making of essential cellular parts such as proteins and neurotransmitters. Ensuring that this chain of command is secure, robust, and well resourced is where the functional neurologist comes in.

The practice of a Functional Neurologist is varied, even skillful. They may draw on a variety of strategies to rouse activity and rebalancing in the nervous system including adjustments in vision, sound, smell, and movement. The effects of these therapies are monitored through measurements of metabolic shifts and affirmed by specific dietary restrictions and prescriptions.

Functional neurology can assist, empower, and drastically improve quality of life for people with a host of challenges, whether it is aging, athletic goals, neurological disturbances, memory loss, creative achievements, or difficulty with focus and concentration. In many ways, functional neurology can be seen as the face of the future of personalized health care at the intersections of simplicity and complexity, growth and healing, medicine and integrative treatment.

References

1. Keystone Chiropractic Neurology. (n.d.) What Is Functional Neurology? Retrieved from http://keystonechiropracticneurology.com/what-is-functional-neurology

Useful Links

Functional Neurology Society
(http://www.functionalneurologysociety.com/index.php)

Parker University Chiropractic Neurology Club
(http://www.parkerneurologyclub.com/)

CHAPTER 20

Testimonials

"I was in a pretty desperate state when I saw Dr. Galyardt. My thyroid was not working, my numbers were really high and I gained over 35 lbs. I had awful mood swings and I was deeply depressed. When we talked I wasn't able to tell him what was wrong because my emotions took over. I couldn't stop crying. Dr. Galyardt asked me, "What I would choose to get rid of first if he had a magic wand." I said, "Depression." I was desperate for change.

My relationships at home were suffering badly. At work I was able to put on a fake smile and hide how badly I felt, but at home all of it came out. Anger out of the blue, deep sadness and emotional ups and downs took a toll on my family. Dr. Galyardt told me about Neurofeedback and how it helps retrain the brain so I could feel good again. I signed up for 40 sessions, two sessions a week. After 2 weeks I already felt a huge difference. My mood swings leveled out. I started to smile and laugh and I didn't have those awful angry outbursts anymore. Everything has gotten better and better with each and every session.

It has been over 4 months since I've finished my neurofeedback sessions and I still feel amazing. I am happy and energetic and I love doing things again. I don't have the urge to hide in my bedroom anymore. I am so grateful for Dr. Galyardt and his wonderful team for giving me my life back.»

— Andi, Fort Collins, CO

"Our daughter Bell started Neurofeedback with Doc Ben, just over a year ago when she was four. She was born with an undiagnosed neurological disorder which has resulted in her inability to walk, or talk, and has significantly affected her cognitive development. We have a dozen other doctors and specialists, none of which, could offer any treatment outside of her therapies. Bell's first Neurofeedback session lasted only six minutes, but the effect was clear. She was alert, and aware of her surroundings, more so than ever before. I cried the entire way home with the painful realization of how disconnected my daughter was with her world.

Within a month every single person associated with our family noticed a difference, even those who were skeptical. It's hard to explain the changes and how significant they were without one knowing where she was before neuro, but that would take to long .

The most notable change was an increase in Bell's endurance and energy level. She went from needing a break from physical activity every 5 to 10 minutes to lasting an entire 45 minute physical therapy session, without any break. Bell's sensory issues which caused her to "stim" all day and limited her the ability to use her hands and interact with her environment, were basically gone. Her perception of her surroundings lined up with her peers. The first time Bell crawled across the living room, from her play room, and into the kitchen I screamed. She never crossed a doorway, let alone roam freely in our house ... she essentially lived in a 5 ft. bubble.

A year later, our sweet daughter Bell is gaining skills in weeks NOT months or years. She is pulling herself to stand and on the verge of walking, she can play all day without becoming exhausted. Her personality is now that of a toddler not a baby. Bell is gaining MUSCLE MASS and strength, and no more sensory issues which resulted in her never using her hands. Doc Ben never made any promises, but he certainly now has given us hope. I cannot wait to see how much neuro helps Bell continue to grow."

– Paula, Fort Collins, CO

"I used to avoid crowds, loud noises and places where there were people because I feared having a panic attack. Once I started on Neurofeedback, I actually felt hope for the first time. It was such a gift to know that I am not losing my mind, and to know that there is a way to retrain the brain to operate on a normal level."

- Laurie, Fort Collins, CO

"When I decided to try Neurofeedback therapy, I was at the end of my rope. I have suffered from depression-like symptoms off and on throughout my adulthood. I had even tried some anti-depressants prescribed by my family

doctor. But I was not happy with the results and worried about the side effects. Yet I had to do something. I was not sleeping well, had no energy, felt overwhelmed. I was also struggling with short-term memory loss and had begun to worry about my performance at work.

The first benefit I experienced with Neurofeedback is the feeling of being in control again. I no longer feel hopeless. The second benefit I experienced is that I started to sleep better. That has made a huge difference in my tendency to overreact to situations. I am no longer as fuzzy-brained or over-emotional.

I am making progress as is shown by subsequent brain maps. I would highly recommend this treatment to anyone suffering from similar symptoms as mine. It's easy and enjoyable. It takes commitment, but is worth it."

– Anne, Fort Collins, CO

"I have tried just about everything offered to relieve the symptoms of chronic fatigue syndrome and fibromyalgia. Neurofeedback Therapy has been by far the most effective. Not only did it reduce my pain by 95%, but it restored my sunny disposition so that I could actually enjoy life once again. For the first time I was being pulled out of the darkness and into wellness."

– Lorna, Loveland, CO

"Anxiety and sleeplessness were becoming increasingly problematic ever since the 'college search' began. I had

brought myself to a scary point of exhaustion. A spiralling pattern of self-destruction trapped me in a somewhat euphoric madness and I was beginning to think it would never turn around. It was time to try something a little out of the box.

Since being treated with Neurofeedback, my abilities have improved have improved a great deal. I am certainly more at ease when it's time to go to bed, and being in public is easier to manage. I still get tired, frustrated and down - but I am able to recognize why I am feeling so, allowing myself to move on.

Medication is now the go-to-treatment of the past. It was a huge struggle skipping along the front lines of the psychiatric world of prescription meds, and I felt fairly little mind-fullness was going into such decisions. Neurofeedback therapy, is far less invasive and risky. I am now able to calmly and effectively set goals and observe consistent personal progress."

– Bob, Fort Collins, CO

Bibliography

**The Mind And The Brain: Neuroplasticity
and the Power of Mental Force**
Jeffrey M. Schwartz, M.D. and Sharon Begley

**Train Your Mind, Change Your Brain: How
a New Science Reveals Our Extraordinary
Potential to Transform Ourselves**
Sharon Begley

Rewire Your Brain: Think Your Way to a Better Life
John B. Arden, Ph.D.

**Soft-Wired: How the New Science of Brain
Plasticity Can Change your Life**
Michael Merzenich

The Brain That Changes Itself
Norman Doidge, M.D.

Brain: The Complete Mind
Michael S. Sweeney

Synaptic Self
Joseph LeDoux

**Functional Neurology for Practitioners
of Manual Medicine, 2nd ed.**
Randy W. Beck, Ph.D.

**My Stroke of Insight: A Brain
Scientist's Personal Journey**
Jill Bolte Taylor, Ph.D.

**The Woman Who Changed Her Brain: Stories of
Transformation from the Frontier of Brain Science**
Barbara Arrowsmith-Young

**Brain School: Stories of Children with Learning
Disabilities and Attention Disorders Who Changed
Their Lives by Improving Their Cognitive Functioning**
Howard Eaton, Ed.M.

Disconnected Kids
Dr. Robert Melillo, DC, DACNB

**Change Your Brain, Change Your Life: The
Breakthrough Program for Conquering
Anxiety, Depression, Obsessiveness,
Anger, and Impulsiveness**
Daniel G. Amen, M.D.

Neuroplasticity and Rehabilitation
Sarah A. Raskin, Ph.D.

**The Body Has a Mind of Its Own: How Body Maps in
Your Brain Help You Do (Almost) Everything Better**
Sandra Blakeslee and Matthew Blakeslee

Keep Your Brain Alive: 83 Neurobic Exercises to Help Prevent Memory Loss and Increase Mental Fitness
Lawrence C. Katz, Ph.D. and Manning Rubin

Phantoms in the Brain: Probing the Mysteries of the Human Mind
Sandra Blakeslee and

The Tell-Tale Brain
V. S. Ramachandran

Brain Maker: The Power of Gut Microbes to Heal and Protect Your Brain – for Life
David Perlmutter

Gut: the inside story of our body's most under-rated organ
Giulia Enders

Spark: How exercise will improve the performance of your brain
By Dr John J. Ratey and Eric Hagerman

The Owner's Manual for the Brain (4th Edition): The Ultimate Guide to Peak Mental Performance at All Ages
By Pierce Howard

Brain Quotes

"The chief function of the body is to carry the brain around."
~Thomas A. Edison

"Tell me what you eat, I'll tell you who you are." ~Anthelme
Brillat-Savarin (1755–1826)

"No diet will remove all the fat from your body because
the brain is entirely fat. Without a brain, you might look
good, but all you could do is run for public office." ~George
Bernard Shaw

"Evolutionarily, sugar was available to our ancestors as
fruit for only a few months a year (at harvest time), or as
honey, which was guarded by bees. But in recent years,
sugar has been added to nearly all processed foods,
limiting consumer choice. Nature made sugar hard to get;
man made it easy." ~Dr. Robert Lustig et al. (R. H. Lustig, et
al., "Public Health: The Toxic Truth About Sugar," Nature
482, no. 7383 (February 1, 2012): 27–29.)

"The brain is a far more open system than we ever
imagined, and nature has gone very far to help us perceive
and take in the world around us. It has given us a brain

that survives in a changing world by changing itself." ~Dr. Norman Doidge (The Brain That Changes Itself)

"As a rule, what is out of sight disturbs men's minds more seriously than what they see." ~Julius Caesar

"Finish each day before you begin the next, and interpose a solid wall of sleep between the two." ~Ralph Waldo Emerson

"At home I serve the kind of food I know the story behind." ~Michael Pollan

"Your brain... weighs three pounds and has one hundred thousand miles of blood vessels. contains more connections than there are stars in the Milky Way.is the fattest organ in your body.could be suffering this very minute without your having a clue." ~Dr. David Pearlmutter (Grain Brain)

"True ignorance is not the absence of knowledge, but the refusal to acquire it." ~Karl Popper

"The brain is a world consisting of a number of unexplored continents and great stretches of unknown territory." ~Santiago Ramón y Cajal

"The asymmery in nature didn't originate with the specialized human mind for art and language; it didn't start late in human evolution; it didn't start in human evolution; it didn't originate with chimpanzees or New World monkeys. It's pre-Jurassic, and so the first evidence is in the fossil

record, even in the placement of molecules." ~Robert Ornstein from The Right Mind 1997

"Brains exist because the distribution of resources necessary for survival and the hazards that threaten survival vary in space and time." John M. Allman (from Evolving Brains, 2000)

"If the human brain were so simple that we could understand it, we would be so simple that we couldn't" ~Emerson M. Pugh (The Biological Origin of Human Values, p. 154, 1977)

"The brain immediately confronts us with its great complexity. The human brain weighs only three to four pounds but contains about 100 billion neurons. Although that extraordinary number is of the same order of magnitude as the number of stars in the Milky Way, it cannot account for the complexity of the brain. The liver probably contains 100 million cells, but 1,000 livers do not add up to a rich inner life. ~Gerald D. Fischback in Scientific American, Sept. 1992

"It is still commonly believed that the human has some completely distinctive characteristics, for example, the possession of language and a high level of artistic and musical abilities. It is my belief that the discovery of dominance [the specialization of the brain] in animals will play a major role in removing these last barriers to the special position of humans." ~Norman Geschwind, 1985

"Men ought to know that from the brain, and from the brain only, arise our pleasures, joy, laughter and jests, as well as our sorrows, pains, griefs, and tears." ~Hippocrates

"If it is mind that we are searching the brain, then we are supposing the brain to be much more than a telephone-exchange. We are supposing it to be a telephone-exchange along with subscribers as well." Sir Charles Sherrington (from Man on his Nature, 1940)

"The brain of modern man, whatever its origins, is better than it need be, and rarely tapped for its true potential." ~Anthony Smith (from The Mind, 1984)

"All beauty comes from beautiful blood and a beautiful brain." ~Walt Whitman (from the preface to Leaves of Grass, 1855)

"Today, when we look at a brain, we see an intricate network of billions of neurons in constant, crackling communication, a chemical labyrinth that senses the world outside and within, produces love and sorrow, keeps our hearts beating and lungs breathing, composes our thoughts, and constructs our consciousness." ~Carl Zimmer (from Soul Made Flesh. The Discovery of the Brain -- and How it Changed the World, 2004)

"The brain is the last and grandest biological frontier, the most complex thing we have yet discovered in our universe. It contains hundreds of billions of cells interlinked through trillions of connections. The brain boggles the mind." ~James D. Watson, from Discovering the Brain

"How can a three-pound mass of jelly that you can hold in your palm imagine angels, contemplate the meaning of infinity, and even question its own place in the cosmos? Especially awe inspiring is the fact that any single brain, including yours, is made up of atoms that were forged in the hearts of countless, far-flung stars billions of years ago. These particles drifted for eons and light-years until gravity and change brought them together here, now. These atoms now form a conglomerate- your brain- that can not only ponder the very stars that gave it birth but can also think about its own ability to think and wonder about its own ability to wonder. With the arrival of humans, it has been said, the universe has suddenly become conscious of itself. This, truly, it the greatest mystery of all." ~V.S. Ramachandran, from The Tell-Tale Brain

"I am a brain, Watson. The rest of me is a mere appendix." ~Arthur Conan Doyle, The Adventure of the Mazarin Stone

"Our brains are obviously capable of astoundingly fast and complex calculations that happen subconsciously. We can't explain them because most of the time we hardly even realize they're happening." - Joshua Foer (Moonwalking with Einstein: The Art and Science of Remembering Everything)

"If you look at the anatomy, the structure, the function, there's nothing in the universe that's more beautiful, that's more complex, than the human brain." - Keith Black (quoted in Discover magazine, April, 2004)

"In order to understand what is meant by the word 'brain' as it is used by neuroscientists, we must bear in mind the evidence that this organ contains in some recorded form the basis of one's whole conscious life. It contains the record of all our aims and ambitions and is essential for the experience of all pleasures and pains, all loves and hates." J.Z. Young (from Philosophy and the Brain, 1987)

"As long as our brain is a mystery, the universe, the reflection of the structure of the brain will also be a mystery."

"Although we tend to think of the brain as a discrete organ - a lump of squidgy tissue - it is better to think of it as part of an elaborate network of nervous tissue that reaches out to every single part of the body." Tim Birkhead (from Bird Sense. What It's Like to Be a Bird, 2012)

"The brain is the organ of destiny. It holds within its humming mechanism secrets that will determine the future of the human race." -Wilder Penfield, The Second Career 1963

"There are two classes of Chiropractors, those who desire to know all they can of physiology, pathology, neurology and anatomy, and those who have an aversion for intelligence, do not want to take effect into consideration, depending only upon an examination of the spinous processes." ~D. D. Palmer